RECOVERY FROM ADDICTION

Recovery From Addiction

A Comprehensive Understanding of Substance Abuse
With Nutritional Therapies
For Recovering Addicts and Co-Dependents

JOHN FINNEGAN AND DAPHNE GRAY

CELESTIAL ARTS
BERKELEY, CALIFORNIA

Reader Please Note: This material has been written and published solely for educational purposes. It should not be used as a substitute for a physician's advice.

Those who need medical attention are strongly recommended to seek out a physician or practitioner knowledgeable in this field and work under his/her direction.

The authors provide this information with the understanding that people act on it at their own risk and with full knowledge that they should consult with health professionals for any help they need.

CELESTIAL ARTS
P. O. Box 7327
Berkeley, California 94707

Quotation from *Love and Addiction*, copyright © 1975 by Stanton Peele and Archie Brodsky. Reprinted by permission of Taplinger Publishing Co., Inc.

Cover design by Ken Scott
Text design and composition by Jeff Brandenburg, ImageComp
Set In Palatino

Library of Congress Cataloging-in-Publication Data

Finnegan, John, 1947-
      Recovery from addiction : a comprehensive understanding of
    substance abuse with nutritional therapies for recovering addicts and co-
    dependents / John Finnegan and Daphne Gray.
          p.   cm.
      Includes bibliographical references and index.
      ISBN 0-89087-599-5 : $9.95
      1. Substance abuse—Diet therapy.   2. Compulsive behavior—Diet
    therapy.   3. Co-dependence (Psychology)—Diet therapy.   4. Nutrition.
    I. Gray, Daphne.   II. Title.
      RC564.29.F56   1990
      616.86—dc20   90-1941
                                                                                CIP
ISBN 0-89087-599-5

First Printing, 1990
0 9 8 7 6 5 4 3
94 93 92

Manufactured in the United States of America

*This book is dedicated
to the thirst for truth
that sets us free.*

Contents

Acknowledgements

First, I would like to give thanks to the power which gave me life in this wondrous gift of creation. While the people who have helped this book come to be are many, my special appreciation goes to my brother Todd, who backed me over the years through thick and thin; to Daphne Gray, my co-author, who made invaluable contributions to this book; and to Kathy Cituk for her insights, editorial and word processing contributions. Others who have made significant contributions are our publisher David Hinds, editors Paul Reed and Carolyn McLuskie. Thanks, as well, to Ken Scott, for his exceptional artwork and cover design. My deep gratitude to my friends and colleagues Lavonne Newell, Brian McDermott, Mimi Calpestri, Robert Natiuk, Dr. Johanna Budwig, John Goodman, Hardy Deering, Lin Winfield, Jeanette Conley, Phil VanKirk, Gilbert Barnes, Bob Walberg, Annie Faye, Bob Quinn, John Kozak, Broda Barnes, M.D., Stephen Langer, M.D., Manfred Mroczkowski, Daniel McBride, and Dolores Rugama. Finally, my special thanks to M.J., whose love and wisdom are reflected in much of the insight and inspiration contained within these pages.

—*John Finnegan*

I wish to thank John Finnegan for inviting my participation in this book, and for the years of friendship and camaraderie we have shared.

I extend special appreciation to our Editor, Carolyn McLuskie, who so artfully melded our two disparate writing styles and types of material, and to Kathy Cituk, for months of total involvement with this manuscript, pampering it through each stage. I also thank Kathy Adams, Ruth Block, Dr. Charles Whitfield, David Pinsley, and Leigh Guilfoyle, for their invaluable insights and contributions.

There are many who aided my personal process, thus making possible much of my contribution. I am indebted to Adult Children of Alcoholics and Codependents Anonymous and their 12-Step programs, to my friend and therapist, Joan Ruderman, to Madolin Winfield, to Beverly Stewart, and to my bodyworkers, Shri Kali Gori and Bevalyn Crawford, who aided me in accessing childhood traumas and working through present as well as deeply buried fears.

My gratitude extends to *A Course In Miracles*, and the *Right Use of Will* books, for inspiration and guidance and for assisting my search for a greater connection with a Higher Power. I owe a great deal to my natal family, who provided the background for "recovery" (which I consider a gift), to my deceased husband, who introduced me to an exciting world that went far beyond my own narrow and parochial concepts, and to my surviving children, Michael, Dawn and Jomo, for accepting me and forgiving my insane (co-dependent) behavior while raising them.

—*Daphne Gray*

Authors' Note

The birth of this book, from conception to publication, evolved into an incredible journey for both of us. Writing is a process itself, as is the "academic" research consisting of reading books, culling and classifying information, interviewing and talking to people, and so on. Perhaps the most profound, however, is the personal research, the growth and change that occurs as you find ways of expressing that which you wish to share. Seeking clarity for the reader, we sometimes find our thoughts are not as clear as we thought they were. Thus begins the process of refining and reworking, not only the expression, but the original idea.

In a book such as this, looking at one's own addictions is a necessary part of the operation. This becomes both painful and joyous, bitter and sweet, tedious and exciting, distressing and hopeful, and—frequently—enlightening.

Co-authoring is also complex, occasionally straining the relationship. But the original respect and love of friends—that caused us to work together in the first place—helped us through hard times—times that bruised our fragile egos and sent us inside to look at our hearts and once again seek honesty and clarity within.

Our deep and sincere desire to make available the vital information in this book helped us through some of the frustrating times. Though there is a proliferation of self help books on the subject of addiction, the essential aspect of proper nutrition and the metabolic causes of addictions is rarely, if ever, approached, especially within the context of other aspects of recovery such as integrating a spiritual program. We leave it to you, the reader, to determine the true value of that which we have imparted.

We also wish to acknowledge each other's contributions and concede that we are not necessarily in agreement on each and every word or idea, but overall have no disagreements on the material presented.

We were delighted to find an editor, Carolyn McLuskie, who so adeptly integrated two sets of information written in different styles into several chapters. Examples of this are found in the Introduction, Types of Addictions and Losing our Connections. Also, bits and pieces are integrated here and there throughout much of the manuscript. Daphne is overall responsible, however, for The Child That Never Was, Getting Help, Rebuilding the Co-Dependent, and the Conclusion.

John, the inspiration for the work, is accountable for all the nutritional and metabolic information. His chapters include The Overview, Metabolic Causes of Addictions and Associated Conditions, Nutritional Therapies, Diet and Recipes (with the help of Kathy Cituk), and Sources of Help and Sources of Formulas.

Our collaboration and effort has been fruitful for us and we hope the end result is fruitful for you, as well.

—*Daphne Gray*
and
John Finnegan

Introduction

Recovery From Addiction presents a comprehensive study of the many factors involved in creating and healing the addictive or alcoholic condition. This book explores the social, economic, and political involvements, as well as the psychological and spiritual dimensions of addiction and co-dependency. It contains some startling new research findings, and attempts to provide complete and up-to-date knowledge on the metabolic basis of addictions. Explained are effective nutritional and medical therapies, a number of which are little known, which help correct the biochemical disorders that lie at the basis of addictions.

Offered here is data on the remarkably powerful effects that certain herbal extracts can have on detoxifying the body, rebuilding the endocrine/glandular and liver function, and strengthening the overall blood sugar/nervous system/metabolic function. The role that yeast overgrowth, or Candida Albicans, can play in the addictive syndrome, is discussed.

In addition to the physical, metabolic causes of addictions, there are cultural and psychological factors. Some ideas on these influences and their relationship to recovery are included, along with a look at 12-Step programs—the most successful method of aiding recovery to date.

Perhaps as basic as the metabolic aspect of addiction is an inner craving for connection, a need to discover one's real self and to feel the power that gives us life. This longing for connection, the need to directly experience significant meaning in life, is often being sought when one succumbs to substance abuse. This aspect—which we call spiritual—is addressed within these pages.

Co-dependency is today being identified as a major problem, woven into the very fabric of our society, within the family, schools, churches, and on the job front. Insights into its origins, its effects, and what to do about it, are offered.

Perhaps most important of all, this book provides solutions— the dramatic, inspiring stories of recovery programs that are working—showing people that they are not powerless victims waiting helplessly for a government agency to come and save them.

Where there is a sincere desire for help, there are real answers. In hearing about successful programs like Daytop, Merritt Peralta Institute, Delancey Street Foundation, and the Betty Ford Center, and the many first hand stories of individuals who turned their lives around, we see that there is much care and help available— that there are real, working answers to these problems. Our lives are not overwhelming burdens, but rather precious gifts, and in honestly facing and handling our challenges we find that a real power exists to guide and free us in our search for true fulfillment.

CHAPTER 1
Overview

Addictions have become one of the most serious social problems facing our world today. Millions of people have died, other millions have suffered serious physical and emotional disease, and countless numbers of families have been shattered by substance abuse. Billions of dollars have been spent on research, therapy and treatment in an attempt to stem the rising tide of addictions to drugs, alcohol, pharmaceuticals and other addictive substances. We have come a long way from the theories that prevailed from the Middle Ages to the early 1900s: the belief that addictions were a moral sin, the cause was a flaw of character and proper treatment was punishment, ridicule and ostracism. Definitive answers are now being developed as to why some people abuse substances while others do not.

Successful programs such as Daytop, Delancey Street Foundation, the Betty Ford Center, and Merritt Peralta Institute, demonstrate that recovery is possible—even for the hardcore addict. They also provide models for other communities concerned with implementing an effective holistic approach which includes job training, education, employment in a supportive environment, a wholesome living situation, rap sessions, and good nutrition.

More and more, police officers are sounding like social workers, expressing the need for a more holistic approach to the drug problem. "A year and a half ago, we were talking about a laundry list of tough-on-crime legislation," said John B. Emerson, Chief Deputy City Attorney of Los Angeles, who leads a legislative subcommittee of the Police Officers Association of Los Angeles County. "But the focus of our panel now is very much on preventive measures. There's been a very dramatic shift."[1]

The same *New York Times* article stated, "The inadequacy of a simple law and order approach to stop the drug problem is obvious when one sees that the number of homicides has nearly tripled in just four years in Washington, and more than half the slayings are drug related.

"New York City jails now hold more than 14,000 drug offenders, seven times as many as in 1980. Nationally, the Justice Department says, arrests for drug abuse violations have increased from 162,177 in 1968 or 112 per 100,000 people, to 850,034 last year, or 450 per 100,000 people. 'In Los Angeles alone last year we made over 50,000 narcotics related arrests, more than all the jail beds in California,' said Larry Goebel, assistant commanding officer of the Dare Program."[2]

A summation of their change in perspective was expressed by Police Chief Fulwood of Washington. "We must recognize the socioeconomic side of this. We've got to have better demand-reduction programs, better treatment facilities. We must build families and communities that have values about murder—that it is not acceptable conduct."[3]

Drug experts now believe that the extreme difficulties faced in treating drug addictions are caused as much by the environment and circumstances of the users as by the biochemical reaction the drug produces. They also believe these new insights offer a measure of hope in developing viable solutions to the drug epidemic that is tearing neighborhoods and families apart in our country today.

"Crack addiction can be treated," said Dr. Herbert Kleber, Deputy to William J. Bennett, Director of the nation's drug policy, in a recent *New York Times* article. However, Dr. Kleber stated, the addict must be given a healthy place in family and social structures to fill these previously unmet needs.[4]

Researchers feel that a primary reason for the high failure rates in outpatient programs is that drug users return to the surroundings and living habits that sent them there in the first place. They do not have the social supports to help them stay away from drugs, and usually lack meaningful, if any, employment. Dr. Kleber and other experts feel that, despite the greater expense, more programs that house the addict should be developed.[5]

Effective programs must help addicts understand the critical need to end all ties to friends and relatives who still use drugs, and help them learn how to establish close friendships with people who do not abuse drugs.

Dr. Michael Scheene, President and Medical Director of the Silver Hill Foundation, a private treatment facility in New Caanan, Connecticut, states, "We have got to get the addicts out of that drug environment. That environment is a morgue."[6]

Sociologists and humanitarian theorists have proposed that many alcoholics/addicts were victims of bad home environments, poverty, poor education, lack of good job opportunities, exploitative and oppressive economic and political conditions, and other problems in the social order. While these are essential factors that must be dealt with, they are not the entire picture, as this theory does not account for the large numbers of addicts populating the professional classes—especially the medical profession, where the addiction rate is four to six times higher than the general population's.[7]

One of the most significant recent breakthroughs in our understanding has been the discovery that addiction is a disease, which has metabolic causes. Between 30 and 40 years ago, Dr. J. W. Tintera, Dr. Abram Hoffer, Dr. Broda Barnes, and others identified these metabolic imbalances as poor adrenal function, low thyroid, low blood sugar and nutritional deficiencies. Today scientific research has added depleted and malfunctioning neurotransmitter, prostaglandin and enzyme systems, as well as inherited genetic malfunction. For example, researchers have recently discovered that the brains of alcoholics produce THIQ, an abnormal chemical that causes alcoholism. All of these factors contribute severe biochemical stresses that lead to substance abuse. When we talk about addictions, we also include the "hidden addictions" to sugar, caffeine, nicotine and pharmaceutical drugs that are only now being understood as truly addictive and can be life-threatening.

What we are also discovering about the addictive personality is a fundamental conflict or adjustment difficulty—not a social-cultural or mental-emotional one, but the basic struggle between spirit and ego. Dr. Carl Jung was probably the first renowned healer in modern times to realize that alcoholism was a disease of the spirit as well as the body. "The craving for alcohol," he wrote, "[is] the equivalent on a low level of the spiritual thirst of our being for wholeness."

Bill Wilson, co-founder of Alcoholics Anonymous, credited the Swiss psychologist as the "first link in the chain of events that led to the founding of AA." Jung had told his patient Roland H., an incurable alcoholic, to face his hopeless state and seek help from a higher power. Roland H. did this, through prayer, meditation and the company of other seekers. To his great joy, he found himself freed from his compulsion to drink. He shared his experience with an alcoholic friend, Edwin T., who, following the same steps, also freed himself from drinking. Edwin T. visited Bill Wilson, who was home drinking, and told him of the change and release that had come into his life.

Wilson later recalled: "Soon after he left me, I became even more depressed. In utter despair, I cried out: 'If there be a God, will He show himself?' There immediately came to me an illumination of enormous impact and dimension."[8]

Wilson's release from the alcohol obsession was immediate and he realized he was a free man. He later had a vision of a society of alcoholics, each identifying with and transmitting his experience to the next. This was the basis for the formation of Alcoholics Anonymous, which has been by far the most successful approach for helping people recover from addictions.[9] AA is a voluntary, worldwide fellowship of women and men who meet to attain and maintain abstinence, and seek sobriety. Because of its anonymous nature, membership records are not kept, but AA does surveys every three years to keep its members and the professional community informed of current trends in membership characteristics. By the end of 1987, there were more than 76,184 AA groups in 114 countries, with about 1,617,296 members.

Today, many are realizing that the addiction problem is multifaceted and needs to be resolved by working in several areas. Many authorities in the field feel strongly that new methods are needed to successfully treat addictions. In "Addiction Recovery Assessed" by Sue Reilly (*San Francisco Examiner and Chronicle*, April 23, 1989), authorities stated that three-fourths of those trying to beat alcohol or other kinds of addictions are not helped by currently available treatments. Dr. Stanley G. Korenman, chief of medical services at the Sepulveda, California, Veterans Administration Medical Center and a member of the staff of the UCLA School of Medicine, said: "The truth is that we are not treating substance abuse successfully. . . . What we need to do is find a way to take a person's addicted cells and return them to their pristine state. We are talking about reversing the chronic changes that occur in brain cells during and after substance abuse. We are talking about regeneration here."

The use of sugar, caffeine, and junk food has broken down many people's normal metabolic perceptions and psyches, opening them up to become users and abusers of hard drugs such as cocaine. Healthy people have feedback mechanisms in their physiology and psyche which warn them that hard drugs are damaging when taken. This self-preserving perception is seriously damaged when excessive amounts of sugar, caffeine or other seemingly innocuous substances are ingested, causing nutritional deficiencies and severe metabolic imbalance. There is more truth than is generally realized in the old adage that use of soft drugs leads to abuse of hard drugs.

An entire society has been created that is malnourished, hyped-up and strung out on caffeine, sugar, preservatives, environmental toxins, alcohol, pharmaceuticals, and fast living. This has caused a predisposition to heavy use of crack cocaine, amphetamines, sedatives, opiates, and other dangerous substances. Parents who have been living on sugar, caffeine, and fast foods are creating a generation of individuals whose bodies and psyches are weakened and susceptible to drug abuse problems.

One of the main reasons that inner city youths have the highest rate of narcotics addiction is because these children also have the highest rates of malnutrition and the greatest percentage of diets filled with empty calorie foods.

In most cases of addiction, there are tremendous nutritional and metabolic disorders which must be corrected before people can have the freedom and ability to choose addiction-free living. In working with disease today, I see six major physical causes of illness: nutritional deficiencies; toxic substances; lack of exercise; infection by yeasts, viruses, bacteria and parasites; and inherited genetic weakness or malfunction, and chronic distress (also called "stress").

The foods we eat simply do not contain the nutrients they once did, due to serious depletion of soils and widespread canning, drying, freezing, storing and refining of foods. This has created severe nutritional deficiencies in the populations of the industrialized nations. Research has shown that a deficiency of a single key mineral or vitamin can make the metabolism so dysfunctional that the blood sugar, glandular, or nervous system malfunctions and induces a craving for sugar or drugs.[10]

Toxins in air, water, and food are a major factor in the breakdown of our physical and mental health today. Increasing numbers of people are developing environmental illnesses. In addition, excessive consumption of sugar, caffeine, marijuana, and alcohol has been found to cause damage as severe as many pharmaceuticals and other drugs. Ingestion of the above-mentioned substances is a main cause of much of today's diseases. Often, people's livers (the body's main cleansing and detoxifying organ) are so damaged that they can no longer break down the toxins. Cirrhosis of the liver ranks fifth as a cause of death for persons aged 45 to 64. At least one-half to two-thirds of the deaths caused by cirrhosis of the liver are directly related to alcoholism.[11] There is a growing body of well-documented evidence showing that liver damage is a main cause of cancer, Candida, arthritis (to a large extent), Epstein-Barr Illness,[12] and environmental illness.

Inherited genetic influences are also a major cause of illness as evidenced by those who inherit constitutions with weak thyroid or adrenal function or those born with a predisposition to produce the alcoholism-causing chemical THIQ.

Accepting the premise that livers are damaged because of toxins, drug abuse and so on, and that weakened livers are a major cause of most illness, what does conventional medicine offer to heal a damaged liver? Basically nothing—except bed rest or a liver transplant, which costs a minimum of $50,000 to $100,000. That is if you can even find a healthy liver, not to mention the trauma and stress of such an operation.

Yet, our bodies can heal most liver disorders with good nutrition and herbs.[13] It takes a little longer than a liver transplant, but many people are reversing life-threatening illnesses by cleaning, rebuilding, and strengthening their livers.[14] How can herbs contribute to a good nutritional program in rebuilding the liver and general health? Herbs provide five different functions:

First, they provide essential nutrients in a synergistically combined form that the body can fully utilize.

Second, herbs provide hormonal precursors—the raw materials that adrenals, thyroid, and other glands use to create hormones, the body's main metabolic regulators. Herbs can increase the body's hormone production and strengthen metabolism.

Third, herbs provide adaptogens and enzymes, substances similar to hormones that strengthen the body and immune system and increase energy and stamina.

Fourth, herbs have antiviral, antibacterial, antifungal, and antiparasitic properties. They kill pathogens without destroying the beneficial flora and without creating Candidiasis, as most antibiotics and antiparasite medications do.

Fifth, herbs have a tremendous capacity to cleanse and pull toxins from the body. For example, Liv.52, one of the formulas recommended in this book—has been found to help the liver eliminate and protect itself from damage by carbon tetrachloride, a powerful carcinogenic poison which causes serious liver damage and immune system breakdown. It also reduces levels of acetylaldehyde.[15]

Two-thirds of our population has heart disease. One of every three people has cancer, and the incidence is increasing exponentially. Much of this cancer is partially caused by toxic substances we ingest and by environmental poisons. But we do have a choice. We can help prevent the poisons from coming in, and we can use herbs and nutrients to cleanse the system. This keeps the liver functioning well so that it does not become over-burdened with toxins, sicken, and break down.

While the most important aspect of a healthy life is a sense of self-worth and an appreciation and love for life, one also needs practical knowledge about what to eat and not to eat, what to do for the condition, and how to heal any existing illnesses. That is one purpose of this book—to share the knowledge and understanding of how the body works and what can be done for it. This book aims to teach the reader how to detoxify addictive substances from the system, regain strength and stamina, and stay drug free, so that life can be enjoyed more fully.

There is another—more subtle—addiction—not substance abuse, but just as devastating to life and the pursuit of happiness. This addiction/dysfunction is called co-dependence. In her best selling book, *Co-Dependent No More*, Melodie Beattie defines co-dependence: "A co-dependent person is one who has let another person's behavior affect him or her, and who is obsessed with controlling that person's behavior." Co-dependents are often the victims of substance abusers: the spouse, child, or other relative or close friend who must cope with having a relationship with an actively-using addict. Co-dependents want to help others, uplift mankind, the world, the underdog, do away with all injustice— but are unable to help themselves. They typically get involved in the lives of those around them and expend great amounts of energy taking care of and trying to solve the problems of others. Their own needs are never as important as someone else's. Low self esteem is at the root of co-dependence.[16]

In this book, we take a look at some of the ways co-depend-ency develops and manifests, as well as how many people are coping with the dysfunction and achieving measures of recovery.

While having an inner experience of truth is the most important part of our lives, being human gives us the chance to enjoy and fulfill the totality of our being. In working with addictions, there are serious aspects of our being that need to be developed and mature, like being practical, responsible, having good values, a willingness to learn, and being honest in our dealings with life.

Most illnesses and addictions are partially caused by a lack of responsibility. All too often, we fail to take responsibility for our lives—responsibility for choosing the kinds of food we eat, the damaging substances we ingest, the kind of work we do, the kinds of relationships we have. Many of us simply do not know how to find happiness. Nor do we have the skills to create a lifestyle that is balanced and fulfilling. We need to find a way to true personal satisfaction and develop identities and ways of living that work within the laws and balance of creation and within our prevailing social milieu.

No nutritional medicine or social activism will have any significant effect in improving our world unless it comes from a real experience of appreciation and reverence for life. There are many forces in society and in ourselves that drive us to self-destructive behavior. Yet, our deepest and truest selves have the power to manifest the beauty and harmony of creation. When we hunger for this truth, it can transform our experience and give us the strength and direction to build our lives anew.

Endnotes to Chapter 1

1. Reinhold, Robert, "Police, Hard Pressed in Drug War, Are Turning to Preventive Efforts" IN *New York Times* (December 28, 1989), page 1.
2. Ibid.
3. Ibid.
4. Kolata, Gina, "Experts Finding New Hope on Treating Crack Addicts" IN *New York Times* (August 24, 1989), page 1.
5. Ibid.
6. Ibid.
7. *Encyclopedia Britannica Research Paper: Street Chemistry and the Dangers of Designer Drugs.*
8. "The Carl Jung-Bill W. Letters," IN *Grapevine* (January 1963).
9. Ibid.
10. Such books as *The Hidden Addiction, Nutrition for Mental Illness, Orthomolecular Medicine for Physicians,* and *Nutritional Influences on Illness.*
11. *Encyclopedia Britannica Research Papers: Alcoholism; The Causes of Alcoholism; Research on the Possible Hereditary Nature of Alcoholism; Physiological Effects of Alcohol; The Problem of Prescription Drug Abuse; The Effects of Cocaine;* and *The Treatment of Narcotics Addicts.*
12. *Chronic Fatigue Syndrome.*
13. *Liv.52: A Monograph,* research paper published by The Himalaya Drug Co., Bombay, India, from over 100 laboratory studies.
14. Ibid.
15. Ibid.
16. Whitfield, C.L., "Co-dependence: Our Most Common Addiction," *Alcoholism Treatment Quarterly*, Vol. 6, No. 1, 1989.

CHAPTER 2

One Woman's Story

"I was working in conference management when I collapsed. The project had required working seven days a week from early morning to late at night. I kept myself going with at least six cups of sweetened coffee a day and a pack of cigarettes, unwinding after work with several drinks, because I was too tired to cook or eat. By the time I literally fell into bed at night, I was so exhausted that sleep was virtually impossible, and the pain radiating throughout my body was so intense that I would lie in bed crying. My blood pressure was dangerously low, and I had pounding headaches that made me dizzy and nauseous for days on end. I suffered from suicidal depression. Every time I closed my eyes, I visualized either stabbing myself with a knife or hanging myself in the shower.

"By the time the project was finished, I seriously wondered if I would be able to go on living. Even the smallest activity was almost too much for me to handle. I had a sense of always being under water, walking against the current. Sheer willpower kept me going. I knew it was time for change, and I made my health my number one priority.

"As fate would have it, I ran into an old friend who gave me a book called *Yeast Disorders*. As I read it, I began to feel there was finally some hope—that each case history could have been mine.

I realized that my life had been a classic setup for yeast. I wasn't breast-fed, so no beneficial floras were implanted in my digestive tract. This led to at least one bout of tonsillitis per year—always treated with penicillin—from the age of four until my tonsils were removed at age 12. My childhood was plagued with chronic bladder problems, skin rashes and viral infections. I slept much more than anyone else I knew. By the time I reached adolescence, my immune system was seriously debilitated and yeast was taking over my intestinal tract. I had a bowel movement only once a week, suffered severe menstrual pain and had several bouts of flu each year.

"At 22, I was taken to the hospital several times with gall bladder attacks. Gall stones a quarter inch in diameter had formed, and when they tried unsuccessfully to squeeze through the minuscule bile duct, I would wind up in the emergency room, writhing in pain. The intern would give me a shot of Demerol. Eventually the pain would subside and I would be on my way. After about four of these visits, the doctors decided to remove my gall bladder. Since I was not aware of any natural way to dissolve gall stones at that time, I let them perform the surgery. Massive doses of antibiotics were administered, of course, and at one point during my recovery, I had such a serious vaginal infection that when I stood up for the nurses to change my bed, the discharge rolled down my legs.

"I never really regained my strength after that surgery, even though a few months later, I left the United States to travel through the Middle East. The years following were made up of high-powered, stressful jobs, requiring a great deal of travel. I was eating a high-carbohydrate vegetarian diet and burnt out time and time again. But I never found out what was wrong, why I had no energy, and why I had one flu and throat infection after another. I tried medical doctors, macrobiotic counselors, naturopaths, chiropractors, acupuncturists, and spiritual healers. Nothing helped.

"I started following the yeast control diet and began taking Chinese herbal formulas right away. For the first two days, I could not get out of bed. On the third day, all the pain in my body was gone. I had forgotten what it was like to not hurt. I lost my craving for coffee and cigarettes almost immediately, and found my body was naturally attracted to the foods that are most nourishing. Although I was feeling much better, I knew I was just beginning the long climb out of the deep, dark hole I had dug for myself.

"I discovered that building one's health after having destroyed it takes a great deal of time, patience, and care. I quit my job and moved in with a friend who was willing to support me for awhile. I started taking a long, serious look at my emotional state, which seemed to have collapsed. The dark depression weighed on my brain, and a feeling of hopelessness and desperation permeated my consciousness. Crying binges were the norm. I read Dr. Stephen Langer's book, *Solved: The Riddle of Illness*. It became evident that low thyroid function had plagued me my whole life, manifested in severe constipation, lack of energy and migraine headaches that made my life miserable. I started on thyroid hormone therapy and felt an immediate response. The black depression lifted, the headaches disappeared immediately, and my metabolism improved. I feel that most people recovering from illness or addiction can heal themselves by using good nutrition, herbs, and supplements. However, some people, like myself, who may have been born with a low thyroid need to use hormonal support in their recovery process.

"My liver had been severely damaged from years of Candida, cigarettes, coffee, alcohol, and drugs, not to mention the everyday toxins that permeate our air, water, and refined foods. I started taking an herbal cleansing formula to help cleanse and rebuild my liver and to rebuild my blood. I took one teaspoon and immediately went to bed for three days with a migraine headache. Shortly after, I turned bright orange—my face, hair and even my eyes. The formula was pulling out deep toxicity and the jaundice lasted for several weeks. I also started taking Liv. 52 and Milk Thistle tablets to help heal my liver.

"I continued taking Chinese herbal products, especially a formula called NuPlus, which is wonderful made into a smoothie with flax seed oil, bee pollen and egg yolks. Pots of herbal teas were always on the stove, and I drank them all day long. Prime Again and adrenal glandular supplements seemed to strengthen my exhausted adrenal glands, and Alpha 20C and Conco strengthened my respiratory and immune systems. I took food complexed vitamins and algae, which also increased my energy, and the addition of mineral supplements to my regimen seemed to relieve the pain that had been developing in my joints. Flax seed oil, GLA, and Beauty Pearls seemed to help my PMS, which had previously turned me into a raging maniac each month.

"My diet had undergone serious changes. Previously, I ate out a lot and downed a lot of fast food, because I was too tired to cook and eat at home. I started eating mostly fresh organic foods with no pesticides, hormones, or antibiotics. I took the time to cook and found my appreciation of life increased. I started to understand how my body works and the importance of the fuel I give it. Whole grains became a favorite food and I found them strengthening and stabilizing, along with lots of fresh vegetables, some fresh fish and poultry. Occasionally I ate some lean red meat. I cannot stress enough how important it is to eat well.

"My insomnia still plagued me until I started making a tea using Chinese licorice, chamomile, and marigold. I found that two cups of this tea taken with several capsules each of Top and Ese provided me with an uninterrupted night's sleep—a pleasure that had been absent from my life for many years.

"I love to walk, so I took long walks in the wooded mountains and along the beach. Fresh air and sunshine do wonders to heal the body and soul. Slowing down and really feeling the movement of my body, the wind in my face, the sun on my shoulders, brought a feeling of peace and stability. Tension and stress melted away with the ebb of the waves, and the salt air soothed my aching heart. I took the time to go inside to experience the essence of my soul, my true self.

"I started to reflect on how I had been living my life. For years I had been taking jobs that were so demanding I'd wind up destroying my health. I started to read about co-dependency and alcoholism and looked back on my childhood. I grew up in a very repressed atmosphere where noisy playing was prohibited, as was any display of strong emotions or creativity. Expression of anger was absolutely forbidden, and I was threatened with physical abuse when I cried. Socializing with neighbors was discouraged, and what went on inside the family was never discussed. My mother, brother and I felt a sense of powerlessness, always 'walking on eggs' so as not to disturb my alcoholic father.

"As a result, I developed a rather strong sense of co-dependency. Everyone else in my life become more important than I was. I lived in such a strong state of denial that I literally felt invisible. Employers loved me. They made outrageous demands, which I cheerfully performed, even if it meant burning myself out working late and on weekends. Asking for help or more pay simply were not options I felt were available to me. I had a deep sense of not being worthy of love or respect. My intimate relationships were disastrous.

"A friend suggested Al-Anon. I felt such an intense resistance to the idea of attending meetings that I knew they would process a lot of my fear, anger, and frustration. I cried all the way through my first meeting and was completely choked up by the end, when newcomers were welcomed to share a few words. I wanted to so badly, but I could only stand there, tears streaming down my face, gesturing with my hands, and mouthing words that squeezed past the lump in my throat to escape as squeaky whispers. Everyone in the room understood. No one laughed at me. Tissues appeared in my hands, and I felt reassuring pats on my shoulders. Thus, I began my 12-step program, which has been a source of inspiration and comfort in my healing process.

"It has been a year since the collapse that literally saved my life. Since then, I have learned much about the workings of my body and the kinds of nourishment it needs. My overall health has strengthened so that I no longer rely on stimulants for energy. The emotional wounds are healing and I am learning to love myself. I no longer act just out of compulsion or duty. I'm learning that my life is a precious gift to be cherished, and that I am a beautiful, loving being worthy of respect and love. A sense of well-being and wonder has returned, and every day is a new beginning in this journey called life."

CHAPTER 3

Types of Addictions

The term "addiction" covers almost all imbalanced and self-destructive behavior, including addictions to power, money, work, suffering, irresponsibility, parasitic behavior, sex, co-dependence, and violence. Substance abuse can create an illusory sense of well-being, but in the long run it severely damages physical and emotional health.

There are underlying metabolic malfunctions common to all substance addictions. Sugar is the foremost addictive substance used today, and several other drugs cause highs through a similar metabolic process. Alcohol is also a simple sugar. Caffeine, psychedelics, amphetamines, and cocaine all temporarily increase the release of sugar into the bloodstream and nervous system. They also duplicate in the nervous system the mood-producing effect of the body's endorphins—chemicals the body produces to transmit messages in the nervous system and brain.

One of the most dangerous and insidious of addictions today is the widespread addiction to pharmaceutical drugs. Millions of otherwise intelligent, responsible people are addicted to chemicals prescribed by well-meaning physicians who often have no idea what damage these high-potency prescription drugs do to a system that is already metabolically imbalanced.

There are many degrees of addiction. Some people are mildly addicted to one or two cups of coffee or a few teaspoons of sugar a day. Others consume two to three quarts of caffeine drinks with a half pound of sugar. A very different approach is needed in dealing with alcohol, heroin, Valium, or other hard drug addiction, as opposed to a milder addiction to a cup or two of coffee or a few cigarettes a day.

People with substance addictions may also have varying degrees of hypoglycemia, borderline low adrenal function, low sexual hormones, low thyroid, B-vitamin and mineral deficiencies, liver malfunction and deficient levels of endorphins, prostaglandins, and neurotransmitters. Severely addicted people can experience extreme depression during withdrawal and develop suicidal tendencies.

Excessive drug use will damage health, weaken the immune system, and contribute significantly to the development of heart disease, cancer, Alzheimer's Disease, diabetes, hypoglycemia, and Candida Albicans overgrowth. Many of these diseases were rare or non-existent 100 years ago. Many children today have inherited weakened immune systems and predispositions to drug abuse from parents who misused drugs and pharmaceuticals.

The abuse of pharmaceutical drugs is one of the most pervasive, yet little-known addictions in the United States today. In 1977, $8 billion was spent on pharmaceuticals—25 percent of it on sedatives and tranquilizers (an estimated 125 million prescriptions to provide 4 billion doses).[1] From May 1976 through April 1977, 54,400 people sought emergency room treatment related to the use, overuse, or abuse of Valium. During that same period, several thousand died from prescription drug overdoses and side effects.

Prescription drugs are not the only culprit. There are more than 300,000 non-prescription over-the-counter drugs, many of which can cause illness and death if misused. Tylenol (acetaminophen) has been found to cause serious kidney damage. In

1977 aspirin was linked to 400 deaths and 17,600 emergency room visits.[2]

Kitty Dukakis, wife of Massachusetts Governor Michael Dukakis, spoke about this little-publicized addiction at the 142nd Annual Meeting of the American Psychiatric Association. Drawing upon her own experience of a 26-year addiction to diet pills which began when her gynecologist prescribed them to her when she was 19, Mrs. Dukakis told delegates there can be "no excuse for the careless prescription of highly addictive tranquilizers and pain killers, particularly when patients who are predisposed to chemical dependency will addict rapidly to these drugs."[3]

Dr. Joseph Pursch, the man former First Lady Betty Ford credits with being the guiding force behind her recovery from pill addiction and alcoholism, calls this disease "the nation's number one health problem."[4]

At a December 5, 1972 hearing on drug abuse in Washington, Wisconsin Senator Gaylord Nelson said that in 1969, the public spent nearly $1 billion on cough and cold remedies, tablets, capsules, drops and sprays. Senator Nelson described these medicines as "mostly useless and sometimes even dangerous."

The Senator added that we want a pill for every ache and pain, for nervous tension, for anxiety, and even for the ordinary stresses and strains of daily living. "In short," he said, "we have become massively addicted to taking drugs whether we need them or not. The result is that we have created a drug culture, and many of the youth of America are simply doing what they have learned from their parents."[5]

There is a growing public outcry against widespread medicating of "hyperactive" children with amphetamines like Ritalin after numerous children on the drug became so depressed that they committed suicide. Parents whose doctors prescribed Ritalin for their children say they were not warned of possible side effects.[6]

A growing number of citizens and physicians are turning from drugs to more holistic healing methods, including psychological support, nutrition, herbs and exercise.

The basic classes of addictive substances are:
- Sugar
- Alcohol
- Nicotine
- Designer Drugs (Alpha Methylfentanyl, also known as White China or synthetic heroin, etc.; MPTP, etc.)
- Psychedelics (LSD, Mescaline, Psylocybin, Ecstasy, MDA)
- Marijuana
- Stimulants (Caffeine, Amphetamines, Cocaine, etc.)
- Depressants (Halcion, Valium, Tranquilizers, Barbiturates, Sleeping Pills, etc.)
- Opiates (Codeine, Demerol, Methadone, Dilaudid, Heroin, Opium, Morphine)
- Steroids (Testosterone, Cortisone, etc.)
- Food Addictions (Bulimia, Compulsive Eating, Food Allergy Addiction Syndrome)

SUGAR

Sugar is the world's most insidious, widespread, and unrecognized addiction and often supports other major addictive processes. People addicted to caffeine or alcohol usually have a strong addiction to sugar as well. Those who succeed in discontinuing addictive drugs, if not using already, usually switch to a combination of nicotine, caffeine, and sugar to compensate for their metabolic imbalances—and wind up perpetuating the self-destructive processes in which they are caught.

Some believe it is inaccurate to classify sugar as an addictive drug. However, one has only to study the metabolic effects of sugar and see what happens when sugar addicts try to stop to realize the potent bite of this invisible addiction. Rarely are people aware that sugar is addictive, or that they themselves are addicted. If they do recognize it on some level ("I just can't pass up a dessert") they usually have no idea what it is doing to their bodies and minds, except perhaps that it produces cavities in the teeth and is fattening.

Two hundred years ago the average American ate less than one pound of sugar a year; today the average U.S. citizen consumes 130 pounds of sugar a year—one third of a pound a day. The first crude sugar was produced from the sap of sugar cane about 2500 years ago. Until the 19th Century, only the wealthy could afford the tiny amounts available. Production soared when slave labor came to the Caribbean in the mid-18th Century, but refined sugar has only been available for about 125 years. World production was about 1½ million tons in 1850. World annual production reached five million tons by 1890; 11 million tons by 1900; 35 million tons by 1950; 70 million tons by 1975—nearly a 50-fold increase in 125 years.[7]

Increased sugar consumption has contributed greatly to the decline of health in our nation. Studies have established that it upsets the body chemistry and destroys the immune system. Excessive consumption of sugar has been conclusively linked to asthma, allergies, arthritis, cancer, heart disease, diabetes, hypoglycemia, Candida Albicans, tooth decay, obesity, headaches, gallstones, osteoporosis and inflammatory bowel disease, among others.[8]

NICOTINE

"According to the Surgeon General, about 1000 Americans die every day from cigarette-related causes. Two fully loaded 747 jumbo jets crashing daily wouldn't kill that many people. Cigarette smoking is the single largest preventable cause of death in the United States, yet every day 3000 kids start smoking—replacing older customers lost to the tobacco industry because they've quit or died."[9]

Next to cocaine, nicotine is considered the most psychologically addicting drug known to man. Next to sugar, and caffeine, it is arguably the easiest addiction to acquire. One of the leading causes of death in the world today is smoking-induced lung cancer.

In 1985, approximately 390,000 deaths were attributable to cigarette smoking. Cigarette smoking is a major cause of cerebrovascular disease (stroke), the third leading cause of death in the United States.[10] Nicotine use greatly increases the likelihood of liver and breast cancer and contributes to heart disease, emphysema, asthma, allergies, headaches, sinusitis, and immune system disorders. Cigarette smoking is now considered to be a probable cause of unsuccessful pregnancies, increased infant mortality, and peptic ulcer disease; to be a contributing factor for cancer of the bladder, pancreas, and kidney; and to be associated with cancer of the stomach.[11] Studies indicate that cigarette smokers are more likely to use other drugs, especially alcohol and marijuana.

The estimated number of compounds in tobacco smoke exceeds 4000, including many that are pharmacologically active, toxic, mutagenic, and carcinogenic. To date, 43 chemicals in tobacco smoke have been determined to be carcinogenic.[12] Inhaling brings nicotine to the brain in seven seconds—half the time it takes a hit of heroin to get to the same place from an addict's vein. The smoker gets a "shot" from each inhalation. At a mere 10 puffs a cigarette, the pack-a-day smoker sends more than 70,000 shots of nicotine to his brain a year.[13]

Nicotine stimulates all body systems, making quitting very difficult. The addition of sugar to commercial cigarettes creates additional problems during the withdrawal process, since smokers may also be sugar addicts. Cigarette smoke cuts the oxygen supply to the eyes, causing a marked inability to visually adapt to darkness, severely limited peripheral vision and tunnel vision.[14]

Women who smoke run twice the risk of delivering a stillborn infant. If the baby does survive, it may be premature and/or smaller, suffer nicotine addiction and withdrawal and have mental and physical impairments. Nicotine reaches the fetus via the mother's blood supply, the infant via breast milk. By 1986, lung cancer caught up with breast cancer as the leading cause of cancer death in women.

In their argument *for* smoking, the authors of *Life Extension* say tobacco use "makes it easier to cope with overstimulation like city noise and overcrowding . . . because nicotine . . . is a stimulus barrier."[15] Like sugar, alcohol, caffeine and narcotics, tobacco desensitizes and is used to make life more tolerable.

Tobacco was first used in the Americas before Columbus. In the mid-16th Century, it was introduced to Spain and Portugal and from there throughout Europe. Its use spread to the Middle and Far East. The tobacco industry has prospered in the United States since colonial times. Prior to the 1900s, nicotine was taken mostly by smoking pipes and cigars, chewing tobacco, and inhaling snuff. The introduction of cigarettes hugely increased tobacco consumption, partly because mass production lowered the price, but also because of extensive advertising by the tobacco industry.

There is some good news, however. Between 1964 and 1985, approximately three-quarters of a million smoking-related deaths were avoided or postponed as a result of decisions to quit smoking or not to start. Each of these avoided or postponed deaths represented an average gain in life expectancy of two decades.[16]

ALCOHOL

Alcohol is the fourth most common addiction in America today, after sugar, caffeine, and nicotine. One standard drink a day can benefit a healthy person by thinning the blood and increasing the metabolic rate. For some, however, even the smallest amount has serious consequences for health and emotional stability. Excessive consumption can cause liver damage, cirrhosis of the liver, hypoglycemia, adrenal exhaustion, kidney or pancreatic damage, ulcers, Candida Albicans overgrowth, nervous system damage, and serious nutritional deficiencies—especially zinc, B vitamins, calcium, magnesium, and other trace minerals.

An *Encyclopaedia Britannica Research Report* entitled "Street Chemistry and the Dangers of Designer Drugs" states the following: "No psychoactive drug is without risks, but most of those concerned with drug regulation in the United States concede that the present system is inconsistent in the way it evaluates those risks. For example, according to the Controlled Substances Act, alcohol should be at the top of the DEA's Schedule 1, which is reserved for drugs whose dangers far outweigh whatever medical utility they may have: it's addictive, destroys brain cells, and causes social destruction, disease, and accidents. According to David Smith, director of the Haight-Ashbury Free Medical Clinic in San Francisco, and others, the ravages of all other drugs combined pale before those of alcohol. Yet alcohol is legal. MDMA and marijuana, on the other hand, are Schedule 1 drugs, controlled as strictly as heroin and more strictly than cocaine, although they don't begin to compare with them in terms of destructiveness."[17]

Several metabolic malfunctions have been identified as the basis of alcohol addiction. Many alcoholics are unable to convert linoleic acids (Omega 6 fatty acids) into gamma linolenic form, crucial in the body's production of prostaglandins. In addition, alcohol consumption depletes the body's already deficient stores of the vital Omega 6 and Omega 3 fatty acids and prevents their conversion into needed prostaglandins.

Alcoholics have been found to have tetrahydroisoquinoline, or THIQ, in their brains. This chemical has a more powerful pain-killing and addictive action than morphine and causes the alcoholic to both crave and be addicted to alcohol. THIQ is also produced in the alcoholic's body from a metabolite of alcohol (acetylaldehyde). For the etiology and therapies for this condition, see the chapter "Nutritional Therapies."

Alcoholics often have endorphin deficiencies, which cause a craving for something to increase their mental-emotional sense of well-being. They often have Candida Albicans and low blood sugar syndrome as well.

Alcohol is very much a part of our heritage. Since its birth, the United States has been a drinking nation. Early 19th Century America was "a nation of drunkards," says history professor W.J. Rorabaugh in *The Alcoholic Republic*.[18] Imbibing alcohol cut across class lines and involved virtually all economic groups, including black slaves, who regularly defied a law prohibiting them from drinking.

The now-institutionalized cocktail hour is an outgrowth of the presidential cocktail party invented by Thomas Jefferson. "Wherever the wealthy congregated, they imbibed great amounts. New York Governor George Clinton honored the French ambassador with a dinner at which 120 guests downed 135 bottles of Madeira, 36 bottles of port, 60 bottles of English beer and 30 large cups of rum punch."[19]

As a member of the aristocracy, Jefferson could afford fine, imported wines that the average citizen could not. Democratic by nature, Jefferson, along with John Calhoun and Henry Clay, promoted the planting of vineyards and enticed the emigration of European vintners to produce wines affordable by all.[20] As a result, America now boasts the world's largest wine vintner (Gallo Wineries in California's Sonoma Valley) and one of the world's largest wine consumption rates.

According to Rorabaugh, per capita annual consumption of distilled liquors exceeded five gallons in 1830 before falling to less than two gallons, where it remains today. (In 1975, the figure was 8.4 liters.) These figures don't include the consumption of beer, hard cider, wine and other fermented beverages. The temperance movement and increased taxation eventually discouraged drinking at the previous high levels.

Recent research has revealed that susceptibility to alcoholism is inversely related to the length of time an ethnic group has been exposed to it. In addition, a culture's reaction to a drug will determine whether the drug becomes an addictive substance. Psychologist Stanton Peale writes: "Studies . . . have shown that Italians, who have a long and settled experience with liquor, do not think of alcohol as possessing the same potent ability to console that Americans ascribe to it. As a result, Italians manifest less alcoholism."[21]

Peale maintains that if a drug is introduced into a culture without respect for existing institutions and cultural practices, and is associated with political repression or rebellion, excessive use will occur. He compares American Indians, in whom chronic alcoholism developed due to the advent of the white man and subsequent disruption of their cultures, with certain rural Greek villages where drinking is so fully integrated into a traditional way of life that alcoholism as a social problem is "not even conceived of." The American Indian has been exposed to alcohol in large amounts for a mere 300 years.[22]

The social costs of alcohol abuse are overwhelming: in 1977, 45 percent of fatal traffic accidents in the United States were attributed to alcohol. Hospital admission rates are increased greatly by alcohol-related accidents and traumas, as well as the many other medical consequences of alcoholism.

Fetal exposure to alcohol is one of the most common causes, and the most preventable cause, of mental retardation in this country. Thus many obstetricians now recommend that pregnant women drink no alcohol—not even one drink.

OPIATES

Opiates include such drugs as codeine, Demerol, Methadone, Dilaudid, heroin, opium, morphine, and fentanyl. They are highly addictive and can change a free, conscious human being into an addict who will commit harmful, immoral, and illegal acts. They can cause liver damage, nervous system damage, and nutritional deficiencies.

The Harrison Drug Act passed in 1914 required prescriptions for narcotics such as opiates which had previously been freely available. In so doing, according to a recent Ford Foundation Report,[23] the act flushed out some 200,000 to 300,000 opiate addicts who descended in droves on physicians' offices clamoring for prescriptions.

Who are the users? This segment of society has been fluid. In 1914 the known opiate population was 60 percent female, 90 percent white, rural and middle or lower class. By 1945, it was 85 percent male and 75 percent white. Since then this addict population has remained 85 percent male and become steadily younger as well as more minority group concentrated.[24]

DESIGNER DRUGS

"It can take years to become addicted to alcohol, months for cocaine, and one shot for fentanyl (a designer drug analogue of morphone and heroin)," recently exclaimed Will Spiegelman, an anaesthesiologist and addiction specialist at Stanford University Hospital.[25]

Designer drugs are the most dangerous of all drugs because of their bizarre, damaging effects on the nervous system. Users can become catatonic and develop constant hallucinations or other forms of insanity. Designer drugs are synthetically produced analogues (molecular relatives) of drugs with similar effects. The laboratory-produced analogues are cheaper than the original drugs, up to 6000 times more powerful, and far more addicting.[26] The DEA says designer drugs are already a billion dollar industry.[27]

Alpha methylfentanyl can be 1000 times more potent than the original (fentanyl). The dosages are infinitesimal and heighten the risk of overdosing. The side effects are harrowing. MPTP, a designer analogue of Meperidine or Demerol, has produced paralysis among some users. The drug actively destroys brain cells and an estimated 100 people have died and more than 400 people in the San Francisco area alone have developed permanent Parkinson's Disease symptoms because the drug damaged neurotransmitters in parts of the brain.[28] Some users were almost totally paralyzed; others suffer stiffness, tremors and seizures.[29]

An estimated 20 percent of California's 200,000 heroin addicts are now using unapproved fentanyl analogues, which include methyl fentanyl and para-fluorofentanyl, other derivatives and the latest and most dangerous 3-methyl fentanyl. The sufentanil and lofentanil derivatives are 2000 and 6000 times stronger than morphine.[30]

"One chemist working eight hours a day for a week can make enough to supply the whole United States for six months and put it in three shoe boxes. There are 2 micrograms in each dose and you can put enough 3-methyl fentanyl on the head of a pin to kill 50 people," explained Robert J. Robertson, Ph.D., former head of the California Division of Drug Programs. He felt the future looked "bleak" and that "we're going to see more neurodegenerative disease and we're going to have more catastrophes like we've had in California with MPTP."[31]

Gene Haislip, deputy assistant administrator of the U.S. Drug Enforcement Administration summed up this growing crisis with, "The designer drug phenomenon, still in its early stages and apparently concentrated in California, has a tremendous potential for causing widespread destruction across the nation. The drugs' potencies are fantastic. Their toxic effects are bizarre and unpredictable—perfectly normal people are being turned into basket cases in a matter of weeks. We have few means of detecting these drugs, either in the body or on the street. And for the first time in history, many people are knowledgeable enough to synthesize powerful narcotics for a few hundred dollars with readily available materials."[32]

PSYCHEDELICS

In the 1960s, many idealistic but misguided people thought psychedelics (LSD, Mescaline, MDA, etc.) were the answer to everything from depression and neurosis to war and poverty. Psychedelics are experiencing a resurgence of use, especially among young people, although the consumption rate is far lower than during their heyday 20 years ago.

One wonders how many times history need repeat itself. Freud declared that cocaine brought peace, happiness, and boundless creative energy, only to find himself and one of his best friends addicted to the drug. During the 1960s, thousands of people seeking enlightenment from psychedelics damaged their nervous systems, freaked out, jumped off buildings, or became psychotic. The newest addition is MDMA (or Ecstasy), which has yet another following that believes love, peace, and happiness can be found in a chemical. Coming down from Ecstasy can lead to serious depression and insanity.

Any substance that greatly increases the stimulation of the nervous system will at the very least deplete the neurotransmitters and create a corresponding depression. At worst, the drug can cause a malfunction in the delicate biochemical pathways and create a drug-induced psychosis. It is a law of physics that applies to all levels of life—every action creates an opposite reaction.

What is needed are foods, nutrients and herbs that nourish, strengthen, and build up the nervous system. And, above all, to see that love and peace are created by how we live, what we live for, and what we seek and see inside ourselves.

MARIJUANA

The Drug Enforcement Agency lists marijuana as the fourth most abused substance in the world after caffeine, nicotine, and alcohol. Studies consistently show that marijuana is both psychologically and physically addictive. A major active ingredient is delta-9-tetrahydrocannabinol (THC). It is most commonly smoked, distributes itself to all the organs, and is almost completely metabolized in the liver. It takes 28 to 56 hours to eliminate half the dose from the body.

Marijuana use may cause adrenal weakness, hypoglycemia, fatigue, lethargy, breakdown of character structure, and a loss of incentive. Marijuana is not as damaging or addicting as other drugs or pharmaceuticals, and its use does not inevitably lead to hardcore drug abuse. However, it impairs health and breaks down ego structure. Some people feel oppressed by their own harsh ego structure and try to free themselves through the use of sugar, marijuana, and other drugs, but the transformation is illusory. Abstinence may cause irritability, nervousness, and insomnia.

Marijuana is a form of hemp that grows wild in most parts of the world. The first written reference to it was in 2737 B.C., in China, and Emperor Shen Nung taught his people the medicinal value of cannabis sativa. It is believed that cannabis was introduced to Western Europe in 500 B.C.

For centuries the plant has been grown both for medicinal uses and for its fiber. It was first cultivated for fiber use in the United

States in 1611, in Virginia. George Washington grew hemp at Mount Vernon in 1765. Some observers believed he was interested in its medicinal and intoxicating qualities as well as its fiber.

In the United States, Extractum Cannabis was considered a medicine and listed as such in the U.S. Pharmacopeia from 1850 until 1942. It was outlawed as a medicine in 1937. While marijuana has been used recreationally since the latter half of the 19th Century, it was not until the 1950s that it became popular with the American middle class and intelligentsia. By the 1970s its popularity had spread to every stratum and age group of American society. In 1970 the Controlled Substances Act classified marijuana as a Schedule 1 drug ("no known medical use"), making possession a misdemeanor and intent to sell, sale, or transfer a felony. Consequently, and perhaps also because of the growing trend to get "clean and sober," the popularity and use of marijuana declined in the 1980s.

STIMULANTS

Stimulants like caffeine, amphetamines, and cocaine can cause severe damage to the nervous system, liver, kidneys, immune system, adrenal glands, heart and circulatory system. Extreme stimulation of the nervous system, adrenal glands, and metabolism creates severe deficiencies of the neurotransmitters, calcium, magnesium, fatty acids, protein, and B vitamins. Heavy users often develop serious mental disorders, including acute paranoia.

Caffeine

More than 100 million Americans start the day with one or more cups of coffee. Many drink five or more cups a day. At 85 to 145 milligrams of caffeine per cup of coffee and 50 to 65 milligrams per soft drink, this is a serious addiction. One or two cups a day won't hurt a healthy person, but excessive use, or even small amounts if the person is weak, ill, or nutritionally deficient, can cause serious health problems.

Caffeine stimulates the central nervous system. When ingested as a beverage, it begins to reach all body tissues within five minutes; peak blood levels are reached in about 30 minutes. Caffeine increases the heart rate and rhythm, affects the circulatory system, and acts as a diuretic. It may elevate blood pressure and raise blood sugar levels. It stimulates gastric acid secretion. It can postpone fatigue and increase alertness and talkativeness.

Withdrawal causes irritability, difficulty concentrating, fatigue, and headaches. Daily use of up to eight cups a day may cause continuous anxiety and depression, upset stomach, chronic insomnia, breathlessness, heart disease, and mild delirium.

Caffeine has been implicated as a major contributing factor in liver damage, hypoglycemia, depleted adrenal function, cysts, breast and other cancers, headaches, ulcers, irritable bowel syndrome, nervous system damage, heart disease, high blood pressure, insomnia, emotional irritability, and increased severity of pre-menstrual syndrome.[33]

It is believed that coffee beans were first grown around 800 A.D. in what is now Ethiopia, where the crushed beans were mixed with fat and eaten as food.[34] Coffee seeds and seedlings were carried to other parts of the world by colonizers, missionaries, and merchant companies. By the 16th and 17th Centuries, coffee drinking had spread to Persia, Turkey, continental Europe, the British Isles, and the Americas.

Coffee is the largest agricultural import of the United States and the second largest commodity in international trade, after petroleum. About one-third of the world's population drinks it. U.S. coffee drinkers comprised 56.6 percent of world consumers in 1980.

Caffeine is also found in cocoa and the kola nut. Its early use, when derived from these substances, was extolled as a cure for exhaustion, dyspepsia, hangovers, and headaches. Caffeine is widely used as a stimulant in cola beverages, which dominate the $13-billion-a-year American soft drink market. Annual per capita consumption of soft drinks 20 years ago was 382.7 12-ounce servings and, according to the National Soft Drink Association, consumption has risen 7.5 percent annually since 1974. This makes soda pop more popular in the United States than coffee or milk.

Caffeine poses serious risks for pregnant women and their fetuses. A research study[35] reported the following: "The average pregnant woman drinks four cups of coffee a day. A study of 16 pregnant women who drank five to six cups of coffee a day showed the following results: eight spontaneous abortions, five stillbirths, two premature infants and one normal delivery." A 1980 FDA drug bulletin warned: "The FDA advises that as a precautionary measure, pregnant and potentially pregnant women be advised to eliminate or limit their consumption of caffeine-containing products."

The Center for Science in the Public Interest advises physicians: "We have carefully reviewed the scientific literature and conclude the consumption of caffeine increases the risk of birth defects and other reproductive problems. We urge you to consider the evidence that implicates caffeine in reproductive problems. We hope you will counsel your patients who are pregnant to avoid caffeine."

What about decaf? Most U.S. coffee manufacturers use chemical solvents to remove caffeine from coffee. Methylene chloride is the most common extracting agent. The use of Trichioroethylene (TCE) as an extracting agent was stopped in July 1975 after the National Cancer Institute found it produced cancer in mice. Both substances are chlorinated hydrocarbons. Some manufacturers now use other methods of extraction, such as water. However, even decaffeinated coffee still contains three percent caffeine.

What happens to that extracted caffeine? Complete with its solvents, it goes straight to the soft drink and pharmaceutical companies for inclusion in colas and drugs.

Amphetamines

Next to designer drugs, amphetamines—such as methadrine, dexadrine, etc.—are the most deadly and damaging of all drugs. People quickly build a tolerance to amphetamines and need increasing amounts to obtain the same effect. The depression that follows amphetamine use, due to depletion of nervous system, glandular and liver reserves, is severe and compels further abuse.

Amphetamines have been greatly misrepresented to the public as safe and beneficial. It is estimated that American soldiers stationed in Britain during World War II consumed 180 million pills of benzedrine. Between 1966 and 1969 the U.S. Army consumed more amphetamines than the combined British and U.S. armies in World War II. In 1971, when production was allegedly being cut back, 12 billion pills were manufactured—60 10-milligram tablets for every person in the United States.[36] Many people became addicted and developed serious physical and mental damage, after their physicians prescribed these seemingly innocuous aids for dieting.

Cocaine

"CITY COULD GO BROKE OVER DRUG" said the headline on the February 21, 1989 issue of the *San Francisco Chronicle*. "Several agencies are devoting a majority of their time and money to the crime, health and social problems created by the drug," the story said. "Last year alone, San Francisco spent about $72 million battling crack—almost $100 for every man, woman and child in the city. The figure is three times the General Fund expenditure for AIDS and roughly matches the budget deficit, which is likely to force cuts in many city services later this year.

"Sixty-six percent of the felony cases filed last year (1988) by the San Francisco District Attorney involved possession or sale of the drug. The crack epidemic created much of the jail overcrowding that now forces crack dealers back to the street."

A recent network TV show stated that drug-related homicide (mostly cocaine) has become the number one killer of children in Washington, D.C.

Cocaine can create serious physiological addiction and sometimes bizarre, destructive actions. A recent TV documentary on the effects of cocaine graphically demonstrated the drug's power. Rats were separated from food and water by an electrified metal grid that gave them severe shocks when they tried to cross. The shocks were so strong that the rats starved to death rather than cross the grid. Yet, once rats had become addicted to cocaine, they would cross the electric grid to get the drug. In other words, addiction to cocaine becomes a more powerful force in the organism than the primary need for food.

Heavy use of cocaine, designer drugs, amphetamines and psychedelics can cause weight loss, anxiety, insomnia, severe depression, paranoia, delusions and hallucinations. There is evidence that consistent use may create a deficiency of norepinephrine stores in the nervous system. The recovery program for cocaine abusers should contain extra use of formulas that support the nervous system.

Cocaine was first used by priests of the Inca Empire who chewed the leaves of the coca bush to enhance their religious experience. In the 1850s a German chemist identified and extracted pure cocaine substance—benzoylmethylecognine—from coca leaves. Use of cocaine in its pure form began in the 1880s when it was given to Bavarian soldiers to counter fatigue and build endurance. Some doctors were using it as a local anesthetic for some surgeries. Sigmund Freud thought it helped his work and published papers extolling its beneficial attributes until reports appeared naming the substance as addicting and also as having caused death by overdose—and until he himself became addicted.

By the early 1900s cocaine was being used in patent medicines and beverages. Coca Cola contained the drug for some 20 years until the government forced the company to delete it from the drink's ingredients in 1906. The Harrison Drug Act of 1914 restricted acquisition of the substance and its use dwindled until the 1960s when drug use again proliferated in U.S. culture.

Earlier classified as a narcotic, cocaine is now legally a stimulant and is occasionally used as an anesthetic for operations on the throat, eyes and mouth because it constricts blood vessels.

Cocaine affects the central nervous system. Its physical side effects are runny nose, eczema around the nostrils and gradual degeneration of the nasal cartilage. Excessive use causes serious deterioration of the nervous system. Death from overdose is possible, with respiratory arrest or heart rhythm disturbances, high fever or seizures. Intravenous ingestion of 1.2 grams may be lethal.

Because of the costs, only wealthy Americans used the drug initially. It became especially popular with sports and entertainment figures. Today cocaine use has spread to all segments of society. An estimated 30 to 60 tons are smuggled into the United States annually, mostly from Colombia. Even drug enforcement officials acknowledge that such estimates are conservative at best.

DEPRESSANTS

In *The Tranquilizing of America*, Dr. Sidney Hook, one of America's foremost philosophers, states: "We have abandoned our old-fashioned values. We have given up our old gods. This nation has turned to tranquilizers almost as a way of life, because people want things to come easily. They no longer want to work hard, to suffer any pain, to feel any stress or anxiety. And what is life without some pain in it? It cannot be all joy.

"We are living in an age of false values, false virtues and false philosophy where the only end seems to be pleasure and gratification. People who take these drugs are lazy. They do not want to take the trouble to find their own center. They are afraid to define their existence. They let a pill do it for them. That's living."

Consumers are led to believe that sleeping pills and tranquilizers are safe and have no damaging side effects. They are often not aware of the dangers of the drugs, nor are they given alternative methods of correcting the problem—such as nutrition, exercise, counselling, visualization, self-love, and personal responsibility.

In a paper published in *Research Communications in Psychology, Psychiatry and Behavior* in 1976, Dr. Louis Gottschalk warned: "We have enough data here to indicate that certain of the benzodiazepines (Valium, etc.) are capable, after a single dose, of significantly disrupting certain kinds of cognitive and/or intellectual functions. Furthermore, this phenomenon outlasts the anti-anxiety effect of these drugs."

Addiction, suicide, nervous system damage, memory loss, and diminished cognitive function are some of the damaging side effects of normal use as well as misuse of tranquilizers.

STEROIDS

"A drug counselor to the National Football League told a state commission that anabolic steroids are the No. 1 problem for athletes. Dr. Forest Tennant told the California Commission on Drugs that 'anabolic steroids are the overriding issue in sports. The use of anabolic steroids is undermining the morale of these people more than cocaine or marijuana.'"[37]

It is estimated that 500,000 teenagers are using anabolic steroids today. Steroids can create debilitating conditions: suppression of normal glandular function, a predisposition to cancer, or immune system disturbances.

People who are serious about building strength and health should learn to use good diet, nutritional supplements, and herbal formulas to attain peak performance. The U.S. Taekwondo Team won four gold, two silver, and five bronze medals in the 1988 Olympics. Many team members said the use of Sunrider Chinese herbal formulas greatly increased their performance and lessened recovery time.

FOOD ADDICTIONS

Bulimia

Many people with bulimia suffer from severe nutritional deficiencies, especially zinc, essential fatty acids, and B vitamins. They often have yeast overgrowth, as well. Also, they may have a low blood sugar and low metabolic rate, which causes them to crave something to pick up their energy.

Many medical researchers, including Dr. Carl Pfeiffer and Dr. Alex Schauss, have had excellent results by providing nutritional support to clear up disturbed eating behavior.

Compulsive Eating

The compulsive eating syndrome is often partially caused by low blood sugar, low adrenal, ovarian and thyroid hormones, nutritional deficiencies, and Candida. People with low blood sugar or insufficient endocrine hormones often eat compulsively because they are subconsciously trying to increase their energy through eating. It has often been observed that both people and animals will get bizarre and compulsive food cravings, eating everything from dirt to sugar, in a subconscious attempt to meet their needs. Candida overgrowth also will drive people to excessive eating. The yeast eats most of the carbohydrates, leaving the person perpetually hungry and undernourished, regardless of how much they eat. Many of my Candida clients have said that, even when they eat a large meal before going to bed, they invariably wake up the next morning to discover that they have lost several pounds during the night and they feel like they are starving.

Food Allergy Addiction Syndrome

People have been found to be addicted to foods to which they are allergic. Often this occurs when people eat the same food continually and have underlying emotional or physical illnesses that are created by the food allergy. Typically, this manifests as depression, irritability, hyperactivity, fatigue, skin disorders, sinusitis, allergies, and digestive disorders.

The most commonly eaten foods that can create this disorder are: soy products, food yeast, wheat and other gluten grains, dairy products, and eggs. People who often eat the same food and have physical or emotional illness would be wise to consider investigating food allergies as contributing to their condition.

Endnotes to Chapter 3

1. Hughes, Richard and Robert Brewin, *The Tranquilizing of America* (New York: Warner Books, 1979).
2. Ibid.
3. *San Francisco Chronicle* (May 7, 1989).
4. Hughs, op cit.
5. Adams, Ruth and Frank Murray, *Megavitamin Therapy* (New York: Larchmont Books, 1973).
6. *Marin Independent Journal* (May 9, 1989).
7. Newbold, H.L., M.D., *Mega-Nutrients for Your Nerves* (New York: Peter H. Wyden, 1975).
8. As documented in such published books as *Lick the Sugar Habit, The Hidden Addiction, Prevention Encyclopedia of Common Diseases, Fats and Oils, Survival of Civilization,* and *Traditional Foods are Your Best Medicine.*
9. University of California, Berkeley, *Wellness Letter,* Volume 6, Issue 7 (April 1990).
10. *Encyclopedia Britannica Report: Smoking and Health.*
11. Ibid.
12. Ibid.
13. Hatterer, Lawrence, M.D., *The Pleasure Addicts* (New York, A.S. Barnes & Co., 1980).
14. *Encyclopedia of Common Diseases.*
15. Pearson, Durk and Sandy Shaw, *Life Extension* (New York: Warner Books, 1982).
16. *Encyclopedia Britannica Research Report: Smoking and Health.*
17. *Encyclopedia Britannica Research Report: Street Chemistry and the Dangers of Designer Drugs.*
18. Rorabaugh, W.J., *The Alcoholic Republic: An American Tradition* (New York: Oxford University Press, 1979).
19. Ibid.
20. Ibid.
21. Peale, Stanton with Archie Brodsky, *Love and Addiction* (New York: Signet, 1975).
22. Small amounts of specially prepared mixtures had been used for certain rituals.
23. Report for the Ford Foundation.
24. Ibid.

25. *Encyclopedia Britannica Research Report: Street Chemistry and the Dangers of Designer Drugs.*

26. Ibid.

27. Ibid.

28. Ibid.

29. Seymour, Richard B. and David E. Smith, M.D., *Drugfree* (New York: Sarah Lazin Books, 1987).

30. *Encyclopedia Britannica Research Report: Street Chemistry and the Dangers of Designer Drugs.*

31. Ibid.

32. Ibid.

33. In such books as *Lick the Sugar Habit, The Hidden Addiction, The Caffeine Book,* and *Megavitamin Therapy.*

34. The historical data on caffeine in this section is derived from "Caffeine Controversy," *Editorial Research Reports* (October 1970).

35. Coulart, Frances, *The Caffeine Book* (New York: Dodd Mead & Co., 1984).

36. Sabbag, Robert, *Snow Blind* (New York: Avon, 1976).

37. "Doctor: Steroids Top Issue for Athletes," IN *Marin Independent Journal* (August 9, 1989).

Chapter 4

Losing Our Connections

Addictions are rampant in our society today. In the United States, there are more than 10 million alcoholics[1] over the age of 18, more than 200,000 heroin addicts, 70 million who are more than 30 pounds overweight, and 10 million pill abusers. Caffeine claims 100 million addicts, nicotine about 35 million. Sugar—considered the "basic addiction" that precedes all others—spans all ages and is probably the least recognized and the most widespread and incalculable. Marijuana and cocaine are also widely abused.

Alcoholism is the oldest and most prevalent addiction in the United States except for sugar, which only recently has been recognized as addicting. Alcoholism has been extensively studied and analyzed, and it is now established that for every alcoholic, the lives of 10 people are dramatically altered due to their relationship to the addicted person.[2] According to John Bradshaw, a noted authority on addictions, 65 million people in the United States are affected by alcoholism. It seems safe to say that all addictions, not just alcohol, cause dysfunction not only for the addicts, but for those who interact with them.

Several cultural factors pressure us into using addictive substances. Many societies and subcultures consider substance abuse very "hip" and "in." Tremendous peer pressure—supported by TV role models and media advertising—is brought to bear on people to smoke cigarettes, have a drink, a coffee or cola, or use other drugs. Young people are often accused of being square or anti-social and are ridiculed and ostracized if they don't go along with the crowd and use whatever the group is using. Among teens and many subcultures, a male is not considered to be a "real man" if he does not use addictive substances.

Another factor contributing to the creation of an addictive society is the eulogizing and romanticizing of drinking and drug cultures by popular literature, television and movies. Winos were glorified in John Steinbeck's *Tortilla Flats*. Bohemians, beatniks, junkies and hippies were romanticized by Jack Kerouac, Henry Miller, William Burroughs, Ken Kesey, and many other writers. The image of the hard-drinking, tough-fighting, heavy-smoking macho man—exemplified by Ernest Hemingway, John Wayne, Clint Eastwood, Mick Jagger, Jack London, and the Marlboro Man—has been held up as a hero and role model for our young people to emulate.

We rarely hear about the immense suffering these people brought upon themselves and others because of their addictions. Both Ernest Hemingway and Jack London became so depressed after ruining their health that they killed themselves. Jack Kerouac also committed suicide. The children and spouses of these people tell us stories of neglect and abuse. Why perpetuate the myth that this is such a great lifestyle? Look at the results in our society today.

Addiction is not a new evil created by Colombian cartels and Jamaican street gangs. Our society has been condoning and promoting addiction to sugar, caffeine, nicotine, alcohol, and other drugs throughout its history. Professional success is the most revered accomplishment in Western society today. This expectation of achievement and excellence is another pressure. Many people studying for exams in school or working at jobs find that, in order to work the long hours and produce the kinds of results that are demanded of them, they have to take stimulants (caffeine, nicotine, sugar, alcohol, amphetamines, etc.). Others rebel against meaningless, oppressive jobs by taking substances to numb out, or create fantasy states that push away the sordidness of dreary, unmeaningful lives.

As we have moved through life without connection to something higher, something beyond everyday existence, materialism has become our focus. We accept that we are physical, emotional, and mental beings. But there is another fundamental aspect to human nature: spirituality. We are spiritual beings, too. Society fails to validate or honor this basic need for spiritual nourishment. Neglect of this dimension creates disharmony—an imbalance in the soul.

The lack of connection to a greater reality leads many to substance abuse or co-dependence. Both conditions feature dysfunctional people suffering from denial, imbalance, low self-esteem, conflict, and disharmony.

There was a time when work was a great source of meaning, happiness, and nourishment in a person's life. Being a farmer, carpenter, nurse, fisherman, or a mother provided a real place and purpose in the cycle of creation. Through their work, they knew the seasons, loved the wind, the rain, and the earth, and helped and were helped by their fellow men and women. Work gave them a sense of freedom, dignity, and self-reliance. It developed the deepest virtues of integrity and character, and was a power that helped draw the breath of their souls in and out of their bodies.

Being a nurse or a healer meant knowing nutrition, cooking, and herbology. They were skilled counselors and practiced the arts of midwifery. They felt and knew the forests, the plants, and the seasons, knew their influences on man, and how to bring balance and harmony into the effects of the extremes of nature and of man's temperament. Tremendous internal strength, self-reliance, and perception were developed.

Today, being a nurse usually means being employed by and subservient to an institution, putting in shifts at a hospital or clinic, and administering drugs that often damage as much as they heal. Statistics show that more people entering a hospital get worse than get better.[3] What effect does administering this kind of therapy have on the nurses who are its purveyors? Does

the powerlessness and meaninglessness of the professions contribute to the fact that doctors and nurses have one of the highest
rates of drug and alcohol addiction in society?

Western medicine's reliance on "expertise" and a symptomatic approach to illness has contributed greatly to an alienation
from the self. We have given up our own authority and come to
rely on experts to diagnose and treat our ills separately: a
dermatologist for a rash, a gynecologist for menstrual problems,
an internist for stomach upset, and so on. The body and its
ailments have become separated from the whole person.

These "imperial professions," as Ivan Illich calls them, encourage dependency on others who "claim monopolies over
certain dimensions of our lives."[4] Each will treat symptomati-
cally, and rarely find out what in our life might cause a change in
bodily function. This trend toward "expertise" has perhaps
peaked as holistic ideas of treating mind, body and spirit as a
totality gain more credibility—and more solid backing from
research. The true healer will encourage personal responsibility
and offer knowledge or advice as a consultant, not as an expert
who "fixes."

Alienation from the self has been scrutinized for decades by
social scientists, psychologists, economists, playwrights, philosophers, and others. Alienation from creative labor is causing
mankind to lose touch with basic human experience. Mass
society has been profoundly affected.[5] The separation from the
self, the lack of a connection with the universe or a higher power
can manifest in addiction, obsession, mania, compulsion, and
preoccupation with numbing the body and shutting down feelings.

More and more psychologists, psychiatrists, ministers, doctors, health care practitioners, and spiritual teachers are seeing
alcoholism and other addictions as "spiritual emergencies."
Stanislav Grof, M.D., former head of Maryland Research Center
and teacher of psychiatry, says: "A deep craving for transcendence is the unrecognized motive behind the need for alcohol or
drugs . . . Intoxication induces a caricature of the transcen-

dental state and a reduction of emotional pain that bear sufficient similarity to the mystical state."[6]

Cardiologist Meyer Friedman, who pioneered the concept of
Type A and Type B behaviors and their effects on the heart,
claims that workaholism occurs because of a lack of spiritual
values. He says materialism is the culprit: we measure worth by
social position and material goods. He further postulates that
lack of belief in a transcendental being causes unhappiness.[7]

The breakdown of the family system is another major cause of
addictions today. It used to be that a son spent a great deal of time
working with his father in whatever trade or business he pur-
sued, and a daughter spent a good deal of her time helping her
parents around the house and with the family business if they
had one. This long contact with parents exerted a great stabilizing and maturing influence on the boundless energy and pas-
sions of youth. It also instilled deep character development, a
sense of responsibility, and mature values. Today, a great many
families have parents that both work or are single parent families. There are very few extended families or even cohesive
nuclear families, and for many young people their peer group is
their most important world.

This is not an advocation of a return to a simple agricultural or
medieval society, for many of these cultures were entrenched in
repressive roles and authoritative structures as well. Rather, it is
a statement that quality time spent with parents and elders is
sorely lacking today and needs to be created within our homes
and society for many of today's problems to be corrected.

Peer groups of young people do not have the values that come
with age, wisdom, and maturity. The rise of large peer group
societies that young people consider to be their most important
source of values, acceptance, and esteem, is occuring for the first
time in history and is having a profound effect on their behavior.

Young people have no experience with the results of sex—
pregnancy, children, economic pressures—so they pursue it
avidly. Their health, strength, and energy seem boundless, so
they pursue drinking and drugs without any of the hindsight

that adults have of the serious physical and emotional damage this can cause. They also have little understanding and appreciation of the value of life, of property, and of economic security, often living recklessly from day to day.

They often feel pursuing a responsible life is useless when the older generation has created a nuclear arms race that could annihilate the entire planet. They are seeing the environment being destroyed and more value placed on material and professional success than on personal peace and fulfillment.

They see their parents using drugs and strung out on everything from sugar and caffeine to tranquilizers, nicotine, and alcohol.

Parents may already have set their children up physiologically for future addiction. Many fetuses are exposed to drugs by their parents' excessive use of alcohol, caffeine, sugar, nicotine, and pharmaceuticals—predisposing them to an acceptance and craving for addictive substances. With very little to emulate and live for and little meaningful time with their parents, many young people often turn to getting high as something more real and honest than the games adult society plays.

The obsessive pursuit of material wealth, exploitative power, professional success, sexual pleasure, and violence has resulted in increasingly aberrant behavior in children. For the first time in history, large numbers of children have become avid consumers of drugs, alcohol, and horror movies, and have themselves become the perpetrators of violent crime, including murder. In 1988, several front-page articles appeared about children who killed other children for sport, or in imitation of satanistic rituals and horror films they saw on TV or in movie theaters. Incidents of this nature are increasing. New support systems for young people deprived of role models, value systems, and emotional support are essential to stem the tide of addiction, crime, and alienation.

Sadly, we live in a society in denial. Although the government says it is waging a war on drugs, in other ways it drives people to substance abuse through its war on life, freedom, and the environment, and by amassing the nation's wealth into the hands of a small, elite group.

Today, for the first time since the Depression, most of the wealth is concentrated in the hands of a few.[8] "You're not going to have enough locks on the doors or police in the street to protect you from a generation of people who are not part of the mainstream of American economic life," said Congressman Thomas J. Downey, who sits on the House Ways and Means Committee and chairs its Subcommittee on Human Resources. In an article which appeared in the *San Francisco Chronicle*, Downey was warning the United States about its future, about what is incubating in a society in which the gulf between the poor and the rich has become a rank and roiling sea.[9] Economist Isabel V. Sawhill of the Urban Institute, a Washington think tank, reports that the number of people living in hardcore underclass areas more than tripled between 1970 and 1980, and the trend seems to have continued in the 1980s.[10] A March 1989 report by the House Ways and Means Committee said: "From 1979 to 1987 the standard of living of the poorest fifth of the population fell by nine percent, while the living standard of the top fifth rose by 19 percent."[11]

The improbability of economic success and independence can lead people to sell drugs as a way of achieving financial success. The severe poverty, oppression, and exploitation of peoples in Third World countries create a drug growing and smuggling economy as the only means to break out of the destitution in which they are stuck.

Denial is not new to mankind, nor to our society. Early invalidation and the subsequent development of low self-esteem, coupled with being raised in a society that fosters denial and encourages addiction, makes it extremely likely that most of us will suffer from dysfunction. It is very likely that dysfunction will be substance abuse or co-dependence—or both. Co-dependence is an addiction, just as devastating to life as addiction to substances. While the alcoholic often dies of cirrhosis of the liver, the co-dependent will die of stress-related diseases.

We become addicts in order to numb ourselves to knowing, to escape the hunger and loneliness we experience in our separation from ourselves. Addiction is often a reaction to the lack of a sense of ultimate purpose in our life.

Like an erupting volcano that releases accumulated pressure and debris and thus creates a new environment, the pent-up disharmony we experience from our denial, from the separation of spirit and will, is finally erupting into an awareness that we are unwhole. With this consciousness that we are incomplete comes the desire and the ability to be healed. In our quest for self-healing, we help heal our planet and society.

That we are ready to make dramatic changes and seek more meaningful lives is demonstrated in part by the fact that mythologist Joseph Campbell achieved national prominence for recognizing the lack of a spiritual dimension in our lives. By showing the connections between all world religions, he illuminated the basic desire in mankind for what he calls the experience of being alive.[12]

A plethora of recent studies and articles describe how the empty lives of "successful" people are leading them to give up high-paying professional jobs. They are recognizing that money and prestige do not bring the happiness they seek. Many find more service-oriented occupations; others live more simply and learn to enjoy nature. We have entered an era in which the institution and the "organization man" have lost prominence. Self-fulfillment is the replacement. Work that offers personal gratification is becoming more appealing than high-paying, high-pressure jobs.

This trend speaks to a desire for connection, for a sense of purpose and of unity with something beyond materialism and prestige. Each of us has the responsibility to live consciously and develop to our highest potential, regardless of the circumstances. Ultimately, it is up to each of us to go beyond oppressive influences, let go of self-destructive ways, and find ways that nourish and fulfill us that will bind us to the power of truth and love that can transform our lives.

Endnotes to Chapter 4

1. Many experts suggest that there may be as many as 20 million.

2. In the PBS TV series *On the Family*, aired in the summer of 1988, John Bradshaw spoke of more recent studies which put the number of people severely affected by an alcoholic at 27.

3. Illich, Ivan, *Medical Nemesis* (National Health Federation).

4. See Keck, Robert L., *The Spirit of Synergy—God's Power and You* (Tennessee: Parthenon Press, 1978).

5. Bradshaw describes our society as "co-dependent, compulsive ... [and] ... full of sexual denial" (op cit.).

6. From "New Age Philosophy on Addictions," IN *The San Francisco Chronicle* (October 13, 1988), an article covering the 1988 International Transpersonal Conference in Santa Rosa, California.

7. "The 'Type A' Doctor," IN *San Francisco Chronicle* (October 19, 1988).

8. Packard, Vance, "Outrageous Fortunes", IN *New Age Journal* (November/December 1988)

9. Salter, Stephanie, "Rich Get Richer, Poor Get Poorer," IN *San Francisco Chronicle and Examiner.*

10. Passell, Peter, "Forces in Society, and Reaganism, Helped Dig Deeper Hole for Poor," IN *The New York Times* (July 16, 1989).

11. Rauch, Jonathan, "Overestimating the Underclass," IN *This World* (July 23, 1989).

12. The PBS TV series of Bill Moyers interviewing Joseph Campbell, *The Power of Myth*, was enthusiastically received and sparked a surge of sales of his already popular books.

CHAPTER 5

The Child That Never Was

How do addiction and co-dependence become ways of life for individuals? The propensity for these illnesses is often rooted in a deep sense of unworthiness. However, this "unworthiness" can be so skillfully repressed that one is totally unaware of it. Indeed, the ego-self may consider unworthiness an extremely unlikely and implausible attribute.

The feeling of being undeserving or unworthy often begins in utero. Studies have shown that if a child is not wanted, the fetus "picks up" that information and enters the world with a deep inner feeling of deprivation, of not being fully loved or accepted. This sense of incompleteness and of not being fully deserving can set one up for abuse on many levels. Self-abuse is common, and addictions are a form of self-abuse. Addiction to abusing others may result as well, as the inherent anger for this state of affairs seeks expression.

Our widespread and culturally accepted ineptness in rearing children is now well documented. We receive more training to operate a cash register or run a race than to handle the monumental task of raising children. Lacking this vital training, most parents often unwittingly invalidate the child's experiences. This confirms to the child that something is wrong with her, that she does not deserve to be loved. Even the planned child with "normal and loving" parents suffers invalidation. It is unusual and rare for a parent to see the child as an individual, separate from the parent's ego. Most of us come from dysfunctional families and perpetuate the dysfunctional system with our own offspring.

Parents tend to get caught up in their image of who they are or wish they were and project this image onto the child, who must then live out this reflection. The child intuits what is expected/ wanted and tries to present to the world a particular image of the family and her role in it by acting out the projection. She is not given the opportunity to develop her own unique self and that real self is rejected, denied and buried.

The person who is predisposed to the addictive process will be one who has been emotionally battered, who was not permitted to be fully expressive, who had to hide and repress real feelings until they were no longer felt. In short, one who had to deny a great deal. Acceptance was there only if the approved reaction or response was forthcoming. The real person, the one under the facade of what was acceptable, is a frightened, lonely child. Somewhere inside millions of adults is a child that never got to be.

Feelings will have been cut off so as to have no more expectations. The ability to receive the body's messages will be deeply buried. There will be unresolved childhood conflicts around autonomy and dependence.

Consider the following scene: Annie's mom and dad are yelling and screaming at each other. Annie is afraid. Daddy slugs Mommy, shouting abusive threats, and slams out of the house. Annie tries to comfort her sobbing mom, who is huddled in a chair. Tearfully, her mom straightens and says: "Don't worry dear, everything is all right."

Or this: Aunt Sara passes out at the dinner table, falls off her chair and lies on the floor. Annie's family ignores the situation—denies it—and tells her: "Nothing is wrong."

These are the people Annie depends on for her very existence. They clothe, feed, house, and teach her. Annie's body and senses tell her something is terribly wrong. But this feeling has just been invalidated. She begins to distrust her own perceptions and thinks: "There must be something wrong with me." Fear quickly follows: "If this is normal, I don't think I can handle bad." Annie lives in dread that something really terrible will happen and she won't be able to handle it.

The need to control becomes primary. Annie quickly learns to suppress inner awareness and feelings. Denial becomes a necessary tool for survival. She must repress anything that might feel scary or like being "out of control." Even strong feelings become equated with losing control.

Annie grows up stuffing her thoughts, feelings, and instinctual behaviors, developing a coat of armor to ward off the pain. She becomes saturated with denial about who she really is, what she really feels, how she really thinks. She doesn't even know what she thinks or feels about anything, because she has learned she can't trust herself. She survives by becoming hypervigilant, quickly surveying all situations, finding out what other people think, what the rules are, what is expected of her, and adapting. She becomes an incredible chameleon, gracefully fitting into any situation. She develops a persona, becoming the person she believes others (especially parents, in the early years) want. She appears to be very well adjusted and capable.

But deep in the core of her being Annie unconsciously carries the feeling of worthlessness, of being somehow different, therefore wrong. She carries shame and a very low self-image. This will cause her to accept many forms of abuse. She may become a workaholic and literally work herself to death in her desperate efforts to please. She may be accident-prone, frequently hurting herself. She may fall into the "women who love too much"[1] syndrome of repeatedly getting into relationships with people who treat her badly. Her insides tell her that is what she deserves. She will be attracted to people who share similar childhood pain and are themselves addicts or co-dependents; people who can only validate the persona, not the frightened, unloved person underneath.

Annie accepts pain and/or punishment stoically, believing that to suffer is her lot in life. She has become totally cut off from feelings and lives in a state of stress. She is afraid of being found out. She believes she is a fraud.

Dr. Lawrence J. Hatterer, a psychiatrist who has worked with addictions for more than 25 years, says that "lack of self-esteem is crucial in addictiveness. The addictive process occurs because the development of the ego and superego are disrupted in childhood . . . the addictive person has excessive expectations of himself but little ability and willingness to discipline himself to perform in ways that enable one to realize them. The frustration that inevitably occurs provokes addictive behavior. The process is inflamed by self-contempt over lack of control of the addictive process and continued poor performance in many aspects of life."[2]

Pursuing her need to feel worthwhile, Annie will be motivated to accomplish "worthwhile" goals. External achievement becomes her ambition, while she neglects the development of any inner sense of self. She will attempt to win the approval of those viewed as worthwhile—usually teachers, parents or other authority figures. Dependent on others for her sense of well-being, she relinquishes control of her life as she strives to please others. Her attempts to become indispensable to others will create the need to outperform everyone and thus the need to be better in order to feel worthwhile at all.

This becomes a never-ending cycle. No matter how much she accomplishes in the external world, Annie will never feel worthwhile. She will be driven to do more, to be more, and still will feel worthless.

Annie will probably be very competent in the eyes of society. She may even believe she is happy, because she is acting like she is "supposed" to act, being the person she thinks others expect her to be. In reality, she is in denial and is totally out of touch with her true being.

Male children will have the same or similar experiences. When the parents fight and dad stomps out of the house, little Jerry comforts his distraught and crying mom. She feels unprotected and vulnerable and may project her need for a man who will take care of things. Jerry unconsciously takes on the role of the man of the house and thereafter tries to take care of and protect his mother; clearly a task he is not capable of. But the need to do it will be there. He will expend great energy and feel responsible, always trying to control events and their outcome. Jerry becomes the little "man of the house," and his parents may reinforce this by bragging about what a "good little man he is."

Jerry becomes a "caretaker" and begins to feel responsible for others' feelings and needs, even anticipating what they may be. Eventually he will feel compelled to solve other's problems. He will find it difficult to let others do for him, feel safest when giving, and feel most alive when there is a crisis in his life—a problem to solve or someone to help. When things go well, he feels bored and insecure and unconsciously creates crises in order to be of use and needed—and simply to feel. His real feelings are deeply buried and inaccessible. The adrenalin rush brought on by a crisis lets him know he is alive. Focusing on the emergency helps distance him from himself. By the time he is a teenager, Jerry needs emergencies.

Society will validate Jerry and Annie for their reliability, their workaholism, their ability to meet crises, to outperform, to handle almost anything.

Parents are not the only ones who may create feelings of unworthiness in a child. Invalidation from an older sibling or an important peer can destroy a child's fragile sense of self. Being teased about one's singing or drawing ability can permanently stifle a child's self-expression and "freeze" an image of incompetence. If the child has only a tenuous sense of accomplishment or ability, the frozen image may remain and the child becomes so convinced she cannot perform in this area that she literally cannot. She grows up handicapped, with missing skills.

Consistent teasing of a child for crying or being afraid can lead to repression of those feelings. The child learns to act as though everything is all right all the time and pushes away thoughts or feelings that contradict this.

These and similar scenarios are repeated time and time again. Each time, feelings of powerlessness and the inability to respond appropriately reinforce the belief that "there must be something wrong with me." Invalidation is cemented and confirmed. Annie and Jerry are taught not to believe what their senses tell them. The result is distrust of their own experience and distrust of other people.

The tendencies for workaholism and caretaking as developed by Annie and Jerry are more common, but not exclusive, to the co-dependent than the practicing addict.[3] These same childhood traumas coupled with genetic, psychological, and social factors will produce other tendencies that lead more directly to substance abuse.

Another child may respond differently to the same invalidation. Instead of becoming overly responsible and addicted to work or caretaking, Liza may become a rebel or dropout. She will fail in school even though she is very bright. She will become the "problem" child. Annie's dysfunction compels her to follow rules and do the right thing, but Liza is untrainable, seeking only to break rules and make trouble. Her focus is to be "different," to attract attention through negative or bizarre behavior, or to hide out, separate herself and be a loner. Daring and compulsive, she will experiment with drugs and other substances at a very early age and likely be an addict by the time she reaches her teens.

Many of us are set up for addiction during pregnancy and/or the birth process itself. If the expectant mother drinks too much, especially during the first three months of pregnancy, fetal alcohol syndrome (FAS) occurs. FAS causes genetic vulnerabilities and susceptibility to alcoholism.[4] If the mother received narcotic pain-killing medications during labor, the child can be born with drugs circulating in its body, numbing it as it enters the world. This predisposes the child to chemical abuse later on.

To go numb is to escape. We do not want to feel, because the pain is too great. All too often, we no longer can feel because we learned not to very early in life. Going numb was often our only survival mechanism: it blocked the disappointment, invalidation, insecurity, and fear.

Society perpetuates the syndrome, validating us for activities that keep us from knowing, being, and feeling who we are. Advertising encourages us to "treat ourselves" to candy, coffee, and cigarette breaks and to reward ourselves with a drink at the end of a work day. For a large percentage of society, drinking liquor has become synonymous with eating a good meal. Companies and corporations contribute heavily to this perception, sponsoring cocktail and dinner parties that encourage excess drinking. Expense accounts support the wooing of potential clients with boozy lunches. "Having fun" always includes plenty of substances that keep us from feeling or thinking.

One may object: "But I feel so great when I'm high. That is the feeling I live for all week. That is my euphoria!" Yes, it may seem so. But the reality is that authentic feeling has been shut down and is inaccessible. The denial of this, the inability and/or unwillingness to access and begin to feel the buried pain and work it through, keeps us stuck with the illusion that we are "fine." The drug-induced euphoria is the closest we can get to experiencing true joy. However, this is far from being in touch with the real self and the experience of wholeness.

When we are encouraged to "get away from it all," to "pamper" ourselves with false euphorias, the implication is that being normal is a drag. We are coaxed and pressured to eat, drink, and smoke in order to be happy, satisfied, and admired. We look outside ourselves for meaning. We are often unable to be alone. We come to need the distractions of a busy or cluttered life, because we are too terrified to look inside. Balance is hard to come by in a world so out of balance. Addiction becomes a coping mechanism, a way out of our pain.

"A person will be predisposed to addiction to the extent that he cannot establish a meaningful relationship to his environment as a whole, and thus cannot develop a fully elaborated life . . . Someone who lacks the desire—or confidence in his or her capacity—to come to grips with life independently . . . (One who is) pessimistic about life and preoccupied with its negative and dangerous aspects.

"Analysis of addiction starts with the addict's low opinion of himself and his lack of genuine involvement in life . . . (The addict-prone) has not learned to accomplish things he can regard as worthwhile, or even simply to enjoy life . . . His lack of self-respect ... (leads) to his belief that he cannot stand alone, that he must have outside support to survive. Thus his life assumes the shape of a series of dependencies, whether approved (such as family, school or work) or disapproved (such as drugs, prisons or mental institutions)."[5]

We will not explore here the particular differences between addiction to substances and addiction to co-dependent behavior. Research has shown the importance of physiological, chemical and genetic factors which predispose and perpetuate addiction. These factors, as well as familial and social experiences, will determine whether the Lizas, Annies and Jerrys move into substance abuse, co-dependent behavior, or both.[6] Both are sicknesses that require special understanding and a focused program for recovery.

Endnotes to Chapter 5

1. In her book *Women Who Love Too Much*, Robin Norwood eluci-dates the syndrome of addiction to relationships that are harm-ful.

2. Hatterer, Lawrence J., M.D., *The Pleasure Addicts: The Addictive Process, Food, Sex, Drugs, Alcohol, Work, and More* (New York: A.S. Barnes and Co., 1980), page 21.

3. For a comprehensive examination of the typical roles that chil-dren from dysfunctional families develop and live out, see: Black, Claudia, *It Will Never Happen To Me* and also Wegsheider-Cruse, Sharon, *Another Chance: Hope and Health for the Alcoholic Family*.

4. People who become alcoholic with their first drink may have been genetically affected in this way. FAS was not discovered until 1970, so there is no way to know how many of today's addicts are victims of this syndrome. FAS produces a small body as well as a small, poorly developed brain. The child is hyperactive, has a short memory, bad humor, and is easily frus-trated and angered.

5. Peele, Stanton and Archie Brodsky, *Love and Addiction* (New York: Signet, 1976), pages 52-56.

6. As more and more substance abusers achieve sobriety in AA, they discover they are still extremely dysfunctional and require other programs such as ACA and/or CODA to complete the process of recovery.

CHAPTER 6

Metabolic Causes of Addiction

... and Associated Conditions

NOTE: For the sake of brevity, formulas and supplements mentioned in this chapter are listed by name only. For detailed descriptions, please see Chapter 7, Nutritional Therapies.

There are seven main metabolic disorders that are partial causes of and associated conditions with addictions: hypoglycemia; liver disorders; endocrine glandular malfunction (mainly thyroid, adrenal, and ovarian); nutritional deficiencies; yeast overgrowth; imbalanced or deficient endorphins, prostaglandins, and neurotransmitters; and the abnormal presence of addictive chemicals like THIQ produced in addictive individuals.

These seven disorders create metabolic malfunctions that can drive people to substances for relief. An optimal recovery program will make an accurate analysis of the individual to determine what is imbalanced and put together the nutritional and medical support necessary to correct the metabolic disorders.

The protocol needs to cover many areas:
1. provide strong metabolic support to the body's basic energy cycles;
2. provide complete nourishing meals;

3. provide replacement hormonal therapy (particularly thyroid) where needed;
4. rebuild the nervous system and replace and help the body produce missing neurotransmitters and endorphins;
5. replace and help the body produce missing enzyme systems such as prostaglandins;
6. strengthen and rejuvenate the glands;
7. cleanse and help heal the liver;
8. build up nutrients which are deficient;
9. cleanse poisons from the system;
10. clear up any existing yeast overgrowth;
11. help the body break down and eliminate toxic addictive substances like acetylaldehyde and THIQ;
12. rebuild any other damaged systems in the body, e.g., immune system, circulatory system, etc.

HYPOGLYCEMIA

There has been so much good material written on hypoglycemia that I will not give an extensive description of this condition. Basically, it is a syndrome and symptom of poor glandular function, imbalanced living, abuse of sugar, alcohol and drugs, nutritional deficiencies, yeast overgrowth, and liver malfunction. The condition has a major deleterious effect on the emotions and nervous system functions, depletes energy, makes one very erratic, and causes often uncontrollable cravings for sweets, alcohol, and drugs. The condition is healed by restoring to balance and good health the underlying causes examined below. See the bibliography for several excellent books on this condition.

LIVER FUNCTION

Liver breakdown results in melancholy, depression, fatigue, and in more severe cases, everything from paranoia to allergies. Hypoglycemia is often caused by an early stage of liver breakdown, and fatigue after a meal is a symptom. Liver damage is the second most frequent cause of the chronic, recurrent yeast condition of Candidiasis, the first being excessive use of antibiotics which destroy the floras that keep yeast under control.

There are five main causes of liver damage: drug use (nicotine, caffeine, alcohol, heroin, cocaine, marijuana, etc.); malnutrition (deficiencies of certain key elements like zinc, the Omega 6 and Omega 3 fatty acids, and B vitamins); Candida, viruses and parasites; environmental poisons (pesticides, lead, formaldehyde from furniture, etc.); and pharmaceuticals and prescription medications.

A doctor I know took medication to lower his blood pressure for a period of one week. It caused such severe liver damage that he spent most of the next year and a half in bed recovering. The symptoms he had developed were severe environmental allergies (he could not even drive on the freeway), serious mental disorientation, inability to concentrate or think, serious Candidiasis, sensitivity to cold weather, food allergies, and fatigue.

The same symptoms appear in people who have had Candidiasis, used excessive amounts of drugs or alcohol, or been exposed to pesticides, and people who were severe vegetarians or fruitarians, which caused severe malnutrition of their livers.

People with yeast conditions fall into two categories. One group develops serious yeast overgrowth after taking antibiotics which killed their beneficial intestinal floras. They recover within weeks by taking digestive floras, killing the yeast, and following a basic diet.

The second group recovers only after adhering to a strict diet, living very carefully, and using a lot of nutritional formulas. But the slightest thing—a little stress, exposure to cigarette smoke, or eating a bit of sweets—can cause a relapse. They get severe Candidiasis all over again, with emotional breakdown, fatigue, and allergies. They go back and forth for years, getting the Candida under control by living very carefully, adhering to strict diets, and using a lot of nutritional formulas; yet they never recover sufficiently to live normally. I believe these people have serious liver damage, and that until they work with formulations to rebuild their liver and glands, they will be subject to recurrent Candidiasis.

The link between melancholy and depression and liver disorders becomes quite obvious when one studies the therapies prescribed for these conditions in homeopathy and traditional European herbal books dating back over the last five to six centuries. Both practices prescribed the same remedy for melancholy and depression, liver deterioration and genital rashes and discharges. In the herbal texts, the term "melancholy" is synonymous with "liver disorders." The diet for liver malfunction recommended for centuries by natural healing doctors and herbalists—in both Eastern and Western traditions—is virtually identical to the established diet for yeast disorders. In short, in some ways we are talking about the same condition. Liver damage causes the weakness in the genital condition, the susceptibility to Candida, rashes, and urinary tract infections. The same liver damage causes mental tendencies towards depression and melancholy, which can lead to suicidal tendencies and paranoia in more severe cases.

The solution is not as simple as killing the yeast. In these conditions, the body does not metabolize carbohydrates properly because of damage to the liver and glands. The carbohydrates stay in the digestive tract and become breeding grounds for yeast. If the body could burn the carbohydrates fully and cleanly, the yeast would not have so many opportunities to grow.

The solution is to kill the yeast, build the floras that control their growth, and restore the metabolic capacity to burn carbohydrates. That means rebuilding the body, the liver, glands and immune system, and correcting nutritional deficiencies. In cases of severe liver damage, this can take months or years. Specific nutrients feed and regenerate the liver and glands, so that as people recover they can slowly introduce more good-quality complex carbohydrates into their diets and be able to metabolize them. There will be a gradual increase of health if they stay with the program and work with it consistently.

Carbohydrate metabolism can be improved by restoring thyroid, liver, and adrenal function, careful use of B vitamins, Calli and Fortune Delight teas, flax seed oil, NuPlus, Prime Again, Action Caps, and zinc. Foods especially good for rebuilding the liver are flax seeds, flax seed oil, beet tops, beets, artichokes, lemon juice (in moderation), Barley Green extract, carrots, greens, whole grains, raw yogurt from good quality milk, organic liver, egg yolks, brewer's yeast and fresh carrot, celery, and beet juice.

Herbs and formulas that help restore liver function are: Liv. 52, Milk Thistle, NuPlus, Calli tea, Sunrider Quinary formula, Km, Alpha 20C, Prime Again, golden seal, vitamin C, carotene, zinc picolinate, ginseng, low dosage B vitamins, Swedish Bitters, and calendula.

The diet for healing liver disorders is almost identical to that for recovery from yeast overgrowth: lots of vegetables, both raw and cooked, fish, fowl and lean meat, small amounts of good-quality fats—especially Omega 3s, small amounts of northern climate fruits, rice, millet, buckwheat, quinoa, other non-gluten grains and potatoes as well as fresh carrot juice for those who do not have hypoglycemia or yeast overgrowth.

ENDOCRINE GLANDULAR FUNCTION

People with long-standing addictions and co-dependents who feel burned out have often weakened their main endocrine glands (thyroid, adrenals, ovaries, and testes). They usually have a depleted adrenal function and often a low thyroid function. Most can restore the normal functioning of their glands through balanced living, good diet, and correct use of herbs, vitamins, and minerals.

Some people need accurate supplementation of hormones either temporarily or permanently. Usually these are people who were born with a weak glandular condition. Some people feel that there is never a need for hormonal support, and that diet, herbs, and vitamins can restore any condition. This has not been my experience, especially with those born with an under-functioning glandular condition. It is one thing to heal an injured leg; it is quite another to try to grow a new leg on someone born with only one.

Correct use of hormones to support an under-functioning gland is a very specialized medical function and must be supervised by a trained medical doctor. It is not within the scope of this book to give a full study of therapy for poor endocrine function; however, since it is a real part of recovery for many addicts, alcoholics, and co-dependents, we will present an overview of this condition.

Good books which elucidate this condition are *Solved: The Riddle Of Illness,* by Stephen Langer, M.D.; *Hypothyroidism: The Unsuspected Illness,* by Broda Barnes, M.D.; *Safe Uses of Cortisone,* by William Jeffries, M.D.; and *Hypoadrenocorticism,* by J. W. Tintera, M.D.

Formulas which can help support or improve thyroid function are: Calli tea, Fortune Delight tea, Km, NuPlus, flax seed oil, B vitamins, Prime Again, Action Caps, Atomidine and other iodine formulas, and dulse seaweed.

Formulas which have been found to help strengthen adrenal function are: NuPlus, Calli tea, vitamin C, B vitamins, zinc, Prime Again, Korean Ginseng, Siberian Ginseng, Bee Pollen, Beauty Pearls, Action Caps, and Adrenal Glandulars.

Formulas which have been found to help strengthen and balance female glandular function are: Beauty Pearls, Prime Again, NuPlus, and Dong Quai. Formulas which have been found to help strengthen male glandular function are: NuPlus, Prime Again, nutritional yeast, B vitamins, Action Caps, and Ginseng.

Flax seed oil is reported to nourish the function of all the endocrine glands.

There are three other ways to improve endocrine glandular function. One is to reduce as much as possible the stresses in one's life. The second is to improve liver function. The liver is involved in producing the precursors to the hormones that the adrenals create. The liver is also a major detoxifier of poisons, and the fewer toxins in the system, the less strain on the glands. It has been observed in many patients that improving their liver function caused a restoration of their endocrine glandular function. The third is, as much as possible, to reduce the intake of toxic substances and foods that create a lot of metabolic waste. One of the main functions of the primary thyroid hormone, and cortisone and adrenaline, two of the main adrenal hormones, is to catalyze the oxidizing and oxygenating metabolic cycles as well as to burn off toxins. The more toxins the glands have to burn off, the greater the strain placed upon them to create more hormones, and the less the hormones are able to perform their other functions of maintaining the health and strength of the organism.

Formulas that help restore liver function are: Liv.52, Milk Thistle, GLA, NuPlus, Calli tea, Km, Barley Green extract, flax seed oil, nutritional yeast, goldenseal, Korean Ginseng, Siberian Ginseng, calendula, and Swedish Bitters.

Foods that are especially good for rebuilding the liver are: beet tops, beets, fresh greens, organic liver, egg yolks, artichokes, and lemon juice (in moderation). Rice, other grains, and potatoes are good for most people, and fresh carrot juice is excellent for those who do not have serious hypoglycemia or yeast overgrowth.

NUTRITIONAL DEFICIENCIES

We have seen that the lack of only one vitamin or mineral can cause a metabolic imbalance that will create a craving for an addictive substance. A fundamental key to this program is the use of vitamins, enzymes, minerals, fatty acids, and herbal extracts to strengthen blood sugar levels and provide good energy and stamina. These will minimize the difficulties of withdrawal and give ongoing metabolic support, making it easier to live a fulfilling life without fatigue or depression, which drives many to some substance for relief.

Nutritional deficiencies and poisons in our foods and environment are the major causes of current illness in the civilized world. According to the U.S. Public Health Service Department, only 3,000,000 people in the entire population can be considered healthy—about 1.5 percent.[1]

The lack of key enzymes, vitamins, minerals, proteins and fats in today's diets is a widespread and debilitating problem affecting the peoples of all industrialized nations.

In December 1945, the United States Soil Conservation Publications reported: "The U.S. produces more food than any other nation in the world. Yet, according to Dr. Thomas Parran, Jr., 40 percent of the population suffers from malnutrition ... Evidently, the food eaten does not have enough of the right minerals and vitamins to keep them healthy.

"Investigators have found that food is no richer in nutrients than the soil from which it comes. Depleted soils will not produce healthy, nutritious plants. Plants suffering from mineral deficiencies will not nourish healthy animals. Mineral-deficient plants and undernourished animals will not support our people in health. Poor soils perpetuate poor people physically, mentally, and financially."[2]

The protein and mineral content of grains dropped 50 percent from the early 1900s to the 1960s and has deteriorated even further today.[3] According to Dr. Walter J. Pories, the soils in 32 states are deficient in zinc.[4] In the 1960s the U.S. Department of Agriculture stated that vegetables and grains had only 50 percent of the magnesium that they had in the early 1900s.[5]

Using whole, unrefined foods prepared without poisonous ingredients and grown on good soils is essential if we want to truly enjoy our lives and not be plagued with physical and mental deterioration.

In the United States today, two-thirds of our population develops heart disease, one-third develops cancer and one-quarter arthritis. One hundred years ago, heart disease was non-existent and the incidence of cancer, arthritis, diabetes, and yeast disorders was minor. Why? What has happened in the last half century to bring such devastating illnesses to some societies and yet leave others untouched? According to many scientific and medical studies, the answer lies in the depletion of critical nutrients due to: soil depletion; shipping, processing, and storage of food; poisons in foods; poisons in the environment; excessive use of sugar, drugs, caffeine, alcohol, etc.; pharmaceuticals; stress; chronic infections; poor assimilation; and lack of exercise.

Many people now realize they are deficient in key nutrients and try to supplement their diets with vitamins, minerals and protein powders. This does not provide all the missing nutrients—for several reasons. First, all vitamin supplements today, whether bought from a large grocery chain store or the most expensive health food store, are synthetic and do not have the same nourishing and healing effects as vitamins in foods. This will come as a great surprise to many people, but all vitamins—except those produced by Grow Company and distributed through its five licensees—are made by five big pharmaceutical houses (Kodak, Hoffman LaRoche, etc.). The pharmaceutical-house vitamins are then sold to different companies to be tableted, bottled, and labeled with their brand names. What about so-called "natural" vitamins like "natural rose hips vitamin C?" True, they are natural. However, according to FDA rules, coal tar and corn syrup are natural and these are the kinds of raw materials from which the vitamins are synthesized.

It has been proven, through hundreds of scientific studies, that synthetic vitamins and minerals have a different molecular structure and do not have the same beneficial effect as nutrients in foods. Now more and more evidence is accumulating which shows that synthetic nutrients in large doses often create imbalance and damage in the organism. There have been many documented cases of people who developed kidney, nervous system and liver damage from mega doses of B vitamins—even doses of 50 milligrams a day. Many formulations contain more than that.

The best way to create a strong, healthy body and mind is to think and live well and eat wholesome foods supplemented by special herbal and whole food extracts and concentrates, with judicious use of vitamin and mineral formulations to give that extra support.

The first and most critical agents needed are those which will replace the addictive substance, while strengthening the body and minimizing withdrawal. The most effective agents found to do this are vitamin C, DL Phenylalanine, Mezotrace, B vitamins, Liv. 52, Km, flax seed oil, gamma linolenic acid, Calli tea, Fortune Delight tea, NuPlus, Prime Again, Milk Thistle extracts, Korean Ginseng, Siberian Ginseng, Action Caps, Swedish Bitters, Beauty Pearls, and mineral formulations.

Liv. 52 is one of the foremost formulas to consider using in the recovery program. With over 300 research studies, it is probably the world's most thoroughly researched plant-based pharmaceutical. It is certainly the most tested and proven formula for improving liver function.

The Sunrider Calli and Fortune Delight teas are especially valuable in replacement therapy. Many people have been able to quit their caffeine, alcohol, and cocaine addictions through use of the Calli and Fortune Delight teas. These teas increase and stabilize blood sugar levels, increase stamina and energy, improve liver function, and are among the most powerful cleansers of body poisons known.

The value of vitamin C in a recovery program is enormous. Many practitioners feel it is the most important nutrient to be used. Besides detoxifying poisons and modifying withdrawal symptoms, this wonderful substance improves immune system functioning, increases oxygenation, and kills free radicals. When taking large doses, it is important to use vitamin C that is buffered with calcium and magnesium. Synthetic ascorbic acid (the vitamin C that is widely used) is highly acidic, and in the non-buffered form it can irritate the digestive tract and leach minerals from the system. Results from recent tests show that food-complexed vitamin C has a far higher assimilation and retention than synthetic vitamin C.[6]

The understanding of the value of flax seed oil is one of the greatest nutritional breakthroughs of this century. This oil has been found to provide the key essential nutrients, the Omega 6 and Omega 3 fatty acids. Now known to be the most essential nutrients needed by the human body, these fats do everything from increase oxygen uptake and utilization to strengthen metabolism, increase nervous system well-being, and provide the precursors for the body's manufacture of prostaglandins, which are increasingly being implicated in addictive behavior and nervous system disturbance.

More and more evidence is showing that often deficiencies in these key nutrients and enzymes causes the metabolic disturbances that lead people to substance abuse.

Many people with addictions have been found to be unable to produce adequate amounts of prostaglandins. These people can use gamma linolenic acid as a source.

Providing strong mineral support is of key importance, especially calcium, magnesium and zinc. Many researchers have found they could reduce withdrawal symptoms by 70 to 80 percent by adding substantial amounts of these minerals to a person's diet.

Calcium and magnesium have essential functions in maintaining nervous system stability. Zinc deficiency has been found to cause everything from the loss of taste to compulsive cravings for sugar and alcohol. Many cases of bulemia, anorexia, and hyperactivity have been cured by taking large amounts of zinc. Chelated zinc picolinate is the most assimilable source of zinc. One of the most remarkable mineral formulations is Mezotrace.

YEAST DISORDERS

Yeast disorders are often a main causative factor in addictions, especially alcoholism, sugar addictions, and eating disorders like anorexia and bulemia. The condition widely known as Candida—a yeast overgrowth in the digestive tract, sinuses, and vaginal area—is widespread. Some authorities estimate that in the United States 60 percent of women and 20 to 30 percent of men develop it in their lifetimes.

Candida and some other species of yeast feed on carbohydrates, and when the body's mechanisms for keeping them under control are thrown out of balance, they will proliferate and cause infections in the tissues. Because these yeasts feed on carbohydrates, an overgrowth will cause intense cravings for, and addictions to alcohol and sweets. Once the infection is under control, the cravings and addictions are greatly alleviated.

An effective program for reducing and controlling yeast overgrowth involves four steps: eliminating simple carbohydrates and reducing complex carbohydrates in the diet; using digestive floras; killing the yeast with goldean seal, Fortune Delight tea, garlic, calendula, methylsulfanomethane or other formulas; and using herbal and nutritional formulas to improve metabolic function, eliminate toxins and rebuild the glands, organs and immune system. (See the bibliography for several excellent books on yeast disorders and nutritional therapies.)

ABNORMAL CHEMICALS: THIQ, EXCESS HISTAMINE

THIQ

One of the greatest breakthroughs in the understanding of alcoholism is the discovery of the presence and function in the brain of abnormal chemicals, some of which have not yet been identified. The most powerful of those identified is an addicting chemical called tetrahydroisoquinoline, or THIQ.

Virginia Davis, a medical scientist, was doing research analysis on fresh human brain when she discovered that brain tissues of alcoholics had high amounts of THIQ. THIQ is closely related in chemical structure to heroin and is very similar in function. The chemical has several unusual properties. It is a painkiller more addicting than heroin. It is produced only in the brains of alcoholics or morphine or heroin addicts by their respective addictive substances. When present in the brain it makes an organism crave alcohol. Rats and monkeys who previously would not touch alcohol preferred it to water after being injected with miniscule amounts of THIQ.

You know the saying: "Once an alcoholic, always an alcoholic." Well, there is a metabolic basis for it. Research proved that once in the system, THIQ stayed there indefinitely. Seven years after being injected with THIQ monkeys were sacrificed and their brains were found to still contain the THIQ. While alive, they had still craved alcohol. This is one of the main reasons why an alcoholic can be dry for 10 or 20 years but go off the wagon completely with one drink.

The addict's body makes THIQ by converting alcohol to acetylaldehyde, then converting a small amount of acetylaldehyde into THIQ. Most people convert alcohol into acetylalde-hyde—which is then eliminated by the body—without creating THIQ.

Candida Albicans yeast also produces a large amount of ace-tylaldehyde. The chemical causes serious damage to the liver and immune system. People whose bodies produce THIQ and who also have yeast overgrowth or Candida Albicans do not necessarily even have to drink. Their bodies can produce THIQ from the acetylaldehyde that the Candida creates. All they need is plenty of carbohydrates to be drunk and sick all the time.

The condition is not hopeless. Medical researchers have found that niacin (vitamin B3) and pantothenic acid (vitamin B5) greatly facilitate the breakdown and elimination of acetylalde-hyde so that it does not end up as THIQ.[7] Dr. H. Sprince and colleagues have published several studies demonstrating the ability of high dose combinations of vitamin C, B1, and the sulfur amino acid cysteine to protect experimental animals from liver-toxic and potentially lethal acetaldehyde. When injected with doses of acetylaldehyde that killed 90 percent of the control animals, the C-B1-cysteine protected animals typically suffered only a 30 percent mortality rate, in comparison.[8] This is one reason why doctors have had such good results when they gave alcoholics B vitamins and a good diet.[9] People have found that some herbal formulas greatly improve their recovery from alco-hol abuse, and I suspect that the herbs help their livers break down the acetylaldehyde.

What is the function of the liver in this process? A strong, functioning liver does most of the functions that neutralize acetylaldehyde so that it doesn't convert to THIQ. People whose liver capacity has been damaged will produce much higher amounts of THIQ. Therefore, one of the main aspects in a successful program for the recovering alcoholic is improving and rebuilding liver function. Foods, vitamins, minerals, en-zymes, and herbs that protect the liver and restore its normal function go a long way towards stabilizing this condition.[10] There have been a number of studies showing that Liv. 52 effec-tively reduces acetylaldehyde blood levels.[11]

Excess Histamine

High histamine levels, also known as histadelia, is a biochemical disorder often associated with addictive tendencies, according to Carl Pfeiffer, Ph.D., M.D. Excessive histamine causes allergic reactions, increased production of mucous and saliva, a tendency to hyperactivity, compulsive behavior, depression, and often suicidal feelings.[12] The individual will unconsciously crave amphetamines, sugar, caffeine, cocaine, heroin, methadone, or alcohol to relieve the pressure caused by an imbalanced body chemistry.[13] Both heroin and methadone have been found to be histamine releasing agents.[14]

Dr. Pfeiffer tested 12 hard-core drug addicts and found them all to be high in histamine. It is also interesting to note that people who are regular drug users often mention that as long as they use amphetamines, cocaine, etc., their allergies clear up and they do not catch colds. Doctors, of course, often prescribe amphetamines to help the allergic patient. The histadelic often develops a yeast disorder as well, and this greatly increases the histamine levels and allergic conditions. Dr. Pfeiffer found that regular use of calcium, manganese, zinc, vitamin B6, methionine, and a good diet help alleviate this condition. After his initial testing of 12 drug addicts, he successfully applied this treatment to over a thousand patients.[15]

Flax Seed Oil, GLA, and many herbs are also helpful in lowering histamine levels, as are thyroid and adrenal support and a good yeast recovery program for those with the associated disorders. Identifying and eliminating foods and environmental toxins to which one is allergic are also critical in healing this condition. Chapter 8—on Nutritional Therapies—has a complete protocol for correcting the histadelic condition.

PROSTAGLANDINS, NEUROTRANSMITTERS AND ENDORPHINS

One of the most exciting and significant areas in modern nutritional science is the study of prostaglandins. These enzymes, which act like hormones, moderate many of the body's essential metabolic processes which govern everything from nervous system and immune system function to one's mental-emotional perceptions.

Blood tests on people who suffered from depression showed that their levels of Prostaglandin E1 were significantly lower than normal. It is theorized that many alcoholics and addicts have an inborn error of metabolism that makes their bodies unable to convert essential fatty acids into needed prostaglandins. An estimated 10 to 20 percent of the Western population is unable to produce adequate amounts of these essential enzymes. It is felt that a deficiency in needed prostaglandins can be a main metabolic factor causing the mental-emotional depression and imbalance that often drives people to addictive substances for relief. Temporary use for 1 to 3 months of gamma linolenic acid will help correct this biochemical malfunction. Increasing one's intake of Omega 3 fatty acids provides the raw materials for one's body to make increased amounts of prostaglandins.

Neurotransmitters are substances the body produces in the nervous system to either inhibit or excite the nerve cells when messages are being transmitted. People who indulge in substance abuse often develop deficiencies and imbalances in their neurotransmitters which can create everything from depression to severe paranoia, and even such serious disorders as catatonic states and Parkinson's Disease.

Endorphins are mood-enhancing neurotransmitter chemicals the body produces to transmit messages in the nervous system and brain. Some endorphins have been found to be 500 times more powerful in their mood elevating effects than drugs such as heroin. Recent research has shown that people with drug dependencies, depression, arthritis, and other conditions are seriously deficient in natural endorphin neurotransmitters.[16]

Endorphins are produced by a combination of processes by the liver, endocrine glands, and nervous system. Genetic defects can cause the body to produce insufficient amounts of endorphins. The condition also can be created through malnutrition, use of drugs, excessive work or living habits, oppressive work and living conditions, emotional shock and traumas, poor emotional and mental attitudes, pesticide and other poisoning, and diseases such as hepatitis, Epstein-Barr (Chronic Fatigue Syndrome), Candida, and other maladies.

There are several ways to increase the body's production of endorphins. A good diet gives the body the raw materials to produce more endorphins. The amino acids D and L Phenylalanine have been shown to produce key nutrients that increase endorphine production. The Chinese Herbal Nervous System Formulas produced by Sunrider are very potent nervous system rebuilders. B and C vitamins, Liv.52, Korean and Siberian Ginseng, Calli tea, Fortune Delight tea, Km, Prime Again, NuPlus, Beauty Pearls, and Action Caps have all been shown to improve sense of well-being by strengthening the liver, glandular, and nervous system functions so that they can produce more endorphins.

Other factors that help are exercise, pursuing a profession and lifestyle that are enjoyable, having good relationships, a healthy living situation, and a sincere and open heart to the experience of life.

Endnotes to Chapter 6

1. Hamaker, John D., *The Survival of Civilization* (California: Hamaker-Weaver, 1982).
2. Ibid.
3. Ibid.
4. Ibid.
5. Ibid.
6. Research studies performed at the following: University of Scranton; University of Missouri; New Jersey College of Medicine and Dentistry; Reims University, France; and the Brain Bio-Center in New Jersey.
7. Hoffer, Abram, M.D., Ph.D., *Orthomolecular Medicine for Physicians* (Connecticut: Keats, 1989).
8. Sprince, H., *et al.*, "Protective Action of Ascorbic Acid and Sulfur Compounds Against Acetaldehyde Toxicity: Implications in Alcoholism and Smoking," IN *Agents & Actions* 5(2): 164-173 (1975).
9. Hoffer, op cit.
10. Werbach, Melvyn R., M.D., *Nutritional Influences on Illness* (California: Third Line Press, 1987).
11. *Liv.52: A Monograph*, published by the Himalaya Drug Co.
12. Pfeiffer, Carl C., Ph.D., M.D., *Nutrition and Mental Illness* (Vermont: Healing Arts, 1987).
13. Ibid.
14. Ibid.
15. Ibid.
16. Phelps, Janice Keller, M.D. and Alan E. Nourse, M.D., *The Hidden Addiction and How to Get Free* (Boston: Little, Brown & Co., 1986).

CHAPTER 7

Getting Help

Finding help and getting support are essential to the healing process, whether one is addicted to substances or to co-dependency. Be persistent in your search—if you have tried and failed, it may be because you have not found the right combination of helpers for yourself and/or because you encounter inner resistance to accepting responsibility for your own healing. This is understandable, as most of us have been taught to turn our healing over to "experts." Perhaps now is the time to change this attitude. We need to participate consciously in our own process—with the help of others—if we are to be truly healed.

Recovery needs to be approached from several perspectives. There is no one thing that does it all. In addition to nutritional supplementation, it may be wise to consider health care providers for the body, therapy, and self-help groups for emotional support and for understanding the roots and process of your addiction. These can be priceless aids to the recovery process. For many, a spiritual program evolves and becomes an integral component in achieving and maintaining perspective.[1]

When setting up your support system, help from people who have successfully worked with addiction problems can be invaluable. There is a great deal of misunderstanding and misinformation on the nature and cause of addictions. Many sincere

79

physicians, nutritionists, and therapists may be willing to work with you but may not have the proper understanding or experience to help you heal this type of problem. Even a well-meaning clergy person can sabotage your process if he or she is ignorant about addictions.

Healing comes from within. It can happen when you open yourself to be healed, and when you participate in the process. On a practical level this means paying attention to yourself, to how you respond to different foods, supplements, people, and ideas. You begin to see yourself as a part of creation, essential to the whole; as a being with a legitimate right and opportunity as a human creature to love, health, and happiness.

You may want to find a practitioner who will help you use the nutritional therapies offered in this book. It is important, however, to listen to your own body as you determine which dosages are correct for you. As you work with yourself, you develop a sense of what is right for you as a unique individual.

Achieving balance takes time. Sometimes your cravings may drive you crazy, and you may want to listen to the addicted part of you that is screaming for substances. A good nutritional consultant will guide you through these crises and help distinguish healthy from unhealthy impulses as you build the former and break down the latter.

Healing means developing a trust that you are basically good and that within yourself there is a wonderful, loving being. At first we tend to be very hard on ourselves and overly critical. Just realize that this is the inner parent and judge, the "old" part of you that has survived by shutting down feelings and developing and impenetrable shell. Be willing to accept yourself with whatever "flaws" you may think you have. Don't be too hard on yourself. If you make a "mistake," observe it, try to learn from it, and go on. Don't beat yourself up about it.

Working with someone who understands cravings and the addictive personality can be especially helpful. If you want nutritional help, find a good nutritionist or holistic doctor who understands the effects of substance abuse and the deficiencies it creates (or the deficiencies that helped create the abuse in the first place) and who will give you the emotional support you need when the going gets rough.

BODY

Many people receive great benefit from bodywork. The body holds all the memories of pain, sorrow, invalidation, and denial that you have suffered. You can heal the emotional traumas in the body and release the unhappy remembrances, while at the same time gaining some perspective on them. Choose a bodyworker who does not simply massage, but who is conscious of the body/mind/spirit connection and is willing to work with you to access repressed traumas and deeply buried feelings.

Movement and exercise are part of the above process. We are often so "busy" that we never make time to take care of the essential body function of exercise. Overcoming addictions is about learning to love and respect yourself; about finding the time to breathe, meditate or pray, exercise, and eat properly. It is about taking care of your spiritual, mental, and physical needs; about finding out that *you* are important and a worthwhile part of the universe.

The survival skills we learned as children growing up in dysfunctional homes included repressing emotions and feelings. The body co-operates: in order to stop the pain, to *not* feel, it tenses. When you are tense, breathing is restricted or nonexistent. In this process, we forgot how to breathe.

In addition, our society's "programming" teaches us that the beautiful body has a flat stomach. Consequently, most of our clothing does not allow proper breathing. You may need to learn how to breathe again. Pay attention to your stomach: is it hard, constricted, knotted? Whenever you become aware of your tummy, let it go soft, breathe deeply, and relax. Consistent practice of this simple "soft tummy" exercise will bring surprising results.

Much addictive behavior and illness spring from a feeling of having no control over one's life. Movement and activity can have an empowering effect on strengthening self-esteem and creating confidence in the ability to change and improve our lives. Taking control of your life and destiny means deciding that you will do what is best for you.

EMOTIONAL SUPPORT

Your friends may change. A difficult and often trying aspect of recovery can be the discovery that it is necessary to move away from some of the people in your life. Giving up your drug of choice is hard enough. Continuing to socialize with people who use makes nearly impossible an already monumental task. When you are solid with your recovery and healing, it may be possible to reconnect with old friends. You may even become an inspiration for them to begin their own healing process. But be careful: don't get caught in a typical co-dependent trap of trying to "fix" others. You are responsible only for yourself.

On the other hand, you are meeting new people, especially if you go to 12-step meetings or participate in group therapy. Because of the fellowship and camaraderie shared, deep friendships often spring forth. One reason the 12-step programs are so effective is that they offer a comfortable social milieu with people who understand what you are going through.

A grieving stage is normal. As with any other life process, when dramatic changes take place and circumstances force you to let go of something or someone dear to you—such as when a death occurs—mourning follows.

As you reclaim your SELF, buried pain and memories may surface, allowing you to work through the anger, resentment, invalidation, and fear that helped lead you to abuse. When you get in touch with the anguish of so many lost moments and experiences, grieving will occur. Also, as you give up habits and patterns that have seemed an integral part of you, grieving will occur. This is normal and appropriate. Please do not try to avoid this stage. You cannot expect to be whole until you allow this process. Some describe this as a rather "bittersweet" experience.

Don't be surprised if you find great resistance to change. Even when we know something is "good" for us, it can be difficult to embrace because it is new and therefore unpredictable or scary. The old, no matter how unhealthy or painful, is still "comfortable" because it is familiar. It takes great courage to embark upon the road to recovery. But the rewards are manifold.

Rebirthing is an option you may consider. It is a process of intentional breathing that can get the body in touch with repressed trauma while at the same time opening the lungs to receive oxygen into the deepest areas—areas that rarely, if ever, get to move out the old, stale air.

Many people find that prayer and/or meditation become an essential aspect of their recovery, helping them to achieve inner serenity and to develop themselves as human beings. Be willing to experiment with several techniques to find which resonates best with you.[2]

Vigorous or aerobic exercise is also recommended. If your body is weak from abuse or poor immune system response, you may need to build a stronger body before engaging in physically demanding exercises. Try walking.

Therapy can be important. You may find validation from a supportive therapist who will recognize your needs for nurturance and not scold or condemn you for the suffering you may have caused yourself and others. A therapist who is also a recovering addict or co-dependent can be especially helpful—assuming he or she has a few years of recovery.

SELF-HELP GROUPS

The need for on-going support groups cannot be too strongly emphasized. Addicts and co-dependents invariably believe they are unique and that no one could possibly understand their particular dynamic. It is an empowering experience to be in a room full of people who share the same problems, emotions, doubts, and mood swings and who suffered the same invalidation. Hundreds of thousands of dysfunctional people are experiencing recovery today in Alcoholics Anonymous-type meetings.

The fellowship of Alcoholics Anonymous (AA) was established in 1935 by two men who had been given up as "hopeless drunks" by their physicians. The program they created worked. They found that asking for help from a higher power, and having a transformational experience, enabled them to stay sober, and to help thousands of others recover and live useful, productive lives. The winning formula was the 12-step program.

Al-Anon was founded in the 1940s by the spouses of alcoholics in AA. In this group, people learned to live with an alcoholic spouse and take care of themselves while they quit focusing on and trying to "fix" the drunk. They adopted the same 12 steps. Ala-teen and Ala-tot were later developments geared to the children of alcoholics.

In the last 5 to 10 years, AA groups have become more and more popular. At the same time, other groups of addicted people used the AA and Al-Anon model to create 12-step programs for their addictions. Overeaters Anonymous was among the first. Today dozens of 12-step groups are springing up all over the country, among them: Narcotics Anonymous, Marijuana Anonymous, Adult Child of Alcoholics Anonymous, Incest Survivors Anonymous, Smokers Anonymous, Sex and Love Addictions Anonymous, Parents Anonymous, Emotions Anonymous, Families Anonymous, Co-Dependents Anonymous, and Cokender Anonymous.

Many of these groups sponsor national conferences in major cities which feature excellent seminars by professionals in the field of addiction. These can be an inspiration and educational tool for the addict or co-dependent. Weekend or all-day workshops led by therapists who specialize in addiction are another option. These intensive sessions offer the opportunity to work through a lot of issues in a condensed period of time and are often an arena for major breakthroughs.

Why and how do these programs work? They stress a simple spiritual approach, with plenty of compassion and understanding for fellow sufferers. The anonymity of all participants is primary, with people giving only their first names when they share and a creed which states that "what you hear within these walls remains here." A camaraderie builds up, often with the very first meeting. This is a safe place to be. The joy of finding people who understand and care is an uplifting and exhilarating experience.

Magical moments can happen in these groups when two different people share a bit of their pasts, or what they are struggling with at the moment. You may not know these people and may never see them again after this meeting. But something each one says triggers a memory in you. You put two and two together and experience a great insight about yourself—why you have a certain characteristic, habit, or attitude. This knowing would not have come about in therapy or anywhere else. Now you have the insight to take to therapy if you wish to pursue it. More importantly, you have learned something about yourself. This can be quite exciting.

There is no "fixing" or "cross-talk" allowed. That is, each person speaks for and about him or herself and does not give advice or promote other groups. People who want advice can ask others to approach them after the meeting. There is a voluntary phone list. Signing it means you are willing to accept program phone calls. In this way, people help each other and know that in a crisis they can call on like-minded people to help them through it. There is no fee for any of the 12-step programs, but the hat is passed at each meeting for donations to cover the costs of rent and free handouts. (Common meeting places are church basements.)

Some people have trouble with the God orientation of the 12 steps. The motto: "Take what you like and leave the rest" helps the wary in their beginning days. Some pretend they have a higher power, calling it something other than God (higher self or nature, for example). Many an atheist and agnostic have successfully worked the steps and achieved recovery. "Surrender to a Higher Power, in fact, consistently leads to expanded, not diminished, responsibility for self and others. AA serves as proof that it is possible to surrender to a Higher Power without giving one's individual power away."[3]

The above 12-step groups have rotating chairpersons selected from the group itself. On the other hand, therapist-led groups, which are usually limited in number of participants, deal with specific addictions. These groups may or may not follow the 12-step format. Frequently, the therapist is a recovering addict or co-dependent. These groups are usually advertised in local publications and neighborhood billboards.

IN-PATIENT/OUT-PATIENT PROGRAMS

You may be saying: "I'm too far gone to follow this outline. I can't even begin." The starting-off point for you could be an in-patient program.

Detox centers are essential for the hardcore addict. They can handle the physical and emotional problems of withdrawal. For example, some alcoholics may have grand mal seizures, suffer mental confusion and hallucinations, or experience drastic blood pressure fluctuations. These symptoms (as well as those of withdrawal from any addiction) need proper care, in order to insure the well-being of the patient.

Residential programs are usually 28 days long. At the outset you will be seen by a physician, a counselor, and a family therapist. A good program will include group and individual counseling, education, stress management and relaxation techniques, a physical fitness regime, and participation in AA or its equivalent (depending on the type of addiction) as well as family treatment and aftercare. Medication to counter withdrawal symptoms and a nutritional regime are an important part of the program.

Aftercare, or "continuing care," is generally a one-year program after discharge. This typically consists of six meetings a week, a personalized continuing care plan and social activities, all offering the recovering addict a lot of support for the process of moving into a useful and productive lifestyle, free of drugs.

If you are in the middle stages of addiction or dependency but still require a structured and fairly intense recovery program, outpatient care can usually be found at the residential facility as well. In a typical program you will meet with a group of six to eight people four times weekly for six weeks. In addition, you will participate in private counseling, group therapy, lectures, films, family treatment and AA, or its equivalent. A one-year continuing care program is available, following the six weeks.

Co-dependents may also become addicts, in the sense of "if you can't lick 'em, join 'em." They will drink with the alcoholic mate and eventually develop a "drinking problem" or become addicted to whatever drug the partner is abusing. In that case, the co-dependent will need to deal first with the substance abuse and later with the co-dependent behavior.

Until recently, the addict has been the "identified patient," and the people in the addict's life simply had to cope as best they could. Today there is a growing awareness that the ones who keep the wheels turning, who shop and cook and clean up for the addict, who make excuses for missed work and smooth over the screw-ups, desperately need help, too. Treatment services for the co-dependent are being added to the curriculum at many detox centers, with both in-patient and out-patient programs. In addition, workshops and seminars are proliferating.

Co-dependent programs help you confront your fear, anger, depression, resentment, frustration—any of the emotional needs you have as one who interacts with a substance abuser. You can get clarity about your own needs, learn how to set and maintain boundaries and get in touch with the wounded child within. A six-day residential program may focus specifically on co-dependency issues, or on the particular issues of the adult child of alcoholic parents.

There are also special programs for other types of problems, such as recovery for the health professional. There may be a monitoring and re-entry program for those who have completed a recovery program.

OTHER THERAPIES

Other healing therapies can be valuable additions in the care of recovering addicts and co-dependents. Acupuncture is a system of traditional Chinese medicine that uses needles to balance the body's energy. Scientific and medical research have established the validity of this mode of treatment. It can help calm the patient during a detoxification crisis and strengthen the body during the long-term recovery process. Acupressure is similar, but uses finger pressure—rather than needles—on specific points to achieve a rebalance of energy. Chiropractic treatment can assist in rebalancing and re-aligning the body.[4]

People occasionally have dramatic responses to homeopathic remedies. However, most need long-term nutritional therapy to heal physical and mental health. Electronic mind balancing machines are being used more frequently by clinics and therapists to treat recovering addicts and some people have been helped greatly by these devices. It is important to use these machines cautiously, as no studies have been done on their long-term effects. One person who used such a device all day long instead of the recommended half hour twice daily had a serious mental and physical breakdown after several months of overuse.

Bear in mind that no one is left to make it alone. If you are willing to seek and work with help, it will be there at every stage.

LONG TERM RESIDENTIAL PROGRAMS

Up to this point we have been speaking to and about individuals who are ready to seek help for their addictions, people who might pick up a book such as this. But what about street addicts, and criminals, whose lives and livings are tied up in the drug scene? Where can they get meaningful help? Prison? Sure, kick it in a prison rehab setting. Then return to your old neighborhood or job, the same people, the same environment. Many are back in jail within 12 hours, often for the same offense. Their treatment program has done little more than cost taxpayers a lot of money.

The strains on society have stretched solutions to the limit. Crime legislation and filling jails with drug abusers and pushers has not brought sought-after results. The drug problem and drug-related crimes increased dramatically in the latter half of the 1980s—to the extent that for the first time in history we have six and eight year-old addicts and pushers.

What are the hopes and possibilities for these hard-core addicts? A handful of surprisingly successful programs have found a solution. What seems to be an essential ingredient in achieving real recovery is being able to live and work in a drug-free social community.

A few long term residential programs offer this. Not just a drug rehab program, but a new life. A total environment for two to four years—long enough to *truly rehabilitate* and reorient a person's life and goals. Education, vocational training, learning to communicate and work with others, plus participating in community service—is helping the so-called "untreatable."

Two highly successful programs, Delancey Street Foundation and Daytop (Drug Addicts Yielding to Persuasion), are demonstrating that accepting personal responsibility and having the opportunity to live and work in an environment that fosters self help can do what law enforcement and prison cannot. Replacing self-destructive cycles with positive experience and self-hate with self-respect (by earning it) is a by-product experienced by participants.

Delancey Street Foundation, headquartered in San Francisco, also has facilities in New Mexico, Los Angeles, New York, and North Carolina. Residents here are defined by society as "unamendable to treatment," with more than 85 percent 10 year heroin addicts.

The average Delancey Street resident has served seven years in prison and has returned to prison three or four times, comes from a poor family, reads and writes at sixth grade level, has no skills, and has never held a job for as long as a year. Yet 70 percent complete a basic two-year course, with many staying the maximum of four years.

There is no staff—no one from the outside who "works with addicts," only residents, working together, in equality. All responsibility and authority is earned. Peers decide on promotions, changes, with all having the opportunity to investigate several vocational options.

Daytop, founded in 1963 by Monsignor William O'Brien, is the oldest and largest drug-treatment program in the United States. It boasts 17 centers throughout New York State, treating 939 in daycare, 900 in residential and 190 outpatient, plus 1350 family members on a weekly basis. Ninety-two percent of its graduates (more than 55,000) are leading self-supporting, drug-free, and responsible lives.

Daytop recently opened facilities in California, Texas, and Florida. It has initiated programs in 40 countries throughout the world.

With an emphasis on doing it yourself and developing usable skills, Daytop and Delancey Street programs generate successful, working citizens. Many become owners of their own companies, some get into real estate or become attorneys, contractors, truckers. In short, their residents learn to live effectively in the dominant American social culture.

Daytop and Delancey Street have become international models of change for substance abusers and criminals. Daytop is funded in part by State and local monies, private donations, client fees, and third party reimbursements. It is staffed by professionals as well as ex-abusers. The program emphasizes honesty, openness, responsibility, and self-help in a tightly controlled setting. Primary to Daytop's rehabilitative process is developing the understanding that drug use signals deep inner conflicts—and these can be overcome.

Delancey Street has succeeded without any government funding. While some financial support comes through donations, much of the funding is internally generated. New residents work in the facility while they receive education and training. Later they work at outside jobs or in one of the center's commercial enterprises and contribute their salaries to the general fund.

In this milieu, ex-addicts, convicts, and prostitutes work together, each person pulling his own weight and developing personal responsibility and a sense of community, much like old-fashioned extended families.

Testimony to the phenomenal success of what has become "far and away to the greatest halfway house in the country, and probably the world."[5] Delancey Street's 500 San Francisco residents began moving into new quarters in early 1990. Situated in downtown San Francisco on the Embarcadero, the project has been hailed a "masterpiece of social design."[6]

While the ground floor of this triangular complex houses retail shops, meeting rooms, a cinema, fitness center, swimming pool, and restaurant, residential units comprise the second floor. An inner courtyard, spectacular views and creative Italian architecture round out the feeling of a cohesive and unique community. The ambience is purposely non-institutional.

Perhaps the most amazing thing about this residential development is that 95 percent of the labor was done by ex-prostitutes, addicts, and murderers who acquired their skills here—with instruction and help from outside professionals.

Between 1971, when Delancey Street began, and January 1990, some 8000 to 10,000 people had changed their lives from no hope to functional citizens. Mimi Silbert, the president and CEO, has been the inspiration and talent that has made this model so successful.

Silbert believes that all people need is a loving, but strict environment and education. Caring about people is holding them accountable, she says. "Our criteria is that you want to change bad enough. We take people everybody thinks are losers. Then with no experience, no funding, just these losers themselves, we develop their strengths."[7]

Needless to say, all of the treatment centers run by these two programs have long waiting lists. However, current expansion is opening their doors to more people. Though Delancey Street now has a new facility, its old one still functions and will continue to do so.

NEW HOPE

The drug problem in the United States appears to be in a transition stage. In 1989 the crack problem reached epidemic proportions, carrying with it deadly implications. For starters, the incidence of crack babies being born was rapidly rising. And

Newsweek (9/11/89) reported crack was wreaking a "ruinous effect on family structure," as more and more women were being implicated. If mother is spending her welfare checks on crack, and selling family possessions for her next hit, what chance do her children have? One result is the occurrence of large numbers of addiction in children under age eight.

The crack problem, along with newer drugs, such as "ice," is clashing with a developing consciousness in mainstream society. Perhaps addiction and its ravishing social consequences is peaking. With every rise there is an inevitable fall.

Several things are happening which point to hope on the horizon. More and more people are reaching out for help, and when it is not forthcoming, they are creating it themselves. Personal responsibility, along with a willingness to share experience for the benefit of others, is a growing phenomenon.

Witness the poor inner city neighborhoods taking responsibility because government help has been too little, too slow, and too encumbered. The people are: organizing block patrols, telling the dealers to get out, organizing anti-drug demonstrations, getting crack houses boarded up, and pushing for job programs to get the kids off the streets. In short, they are taking the matter into their own hands and forcing solutions.

We have already mentioned the growing success of new approaches to drug cure as manifested at Delancey Street and Daytop. There is also a proliferation of detox centers and both in- and out-patient programs. The AA model is succeeding as never before. If a meeting is needed in a community, someone organizes one, whether it be AA, Al-Anon, Coda, NA—whatever. And when that one gets too big, another is created. All one needs to do is find a room to rent (passing the hat should pay for it) and contact the national office. Information packets are sent, and you are on your way. If your group isn't listed in the phone directory, contact AA, they can usually refer you.

Consciousness that addiction is a disease and not a moral sin or character defect is rising. Even the health insurance companies are finally helping to pay for recovery programs.

The phenomenal success of the Betty Ford Center should be mentioned. This is another example of a person who got well and was so thankful that she wanted to help others. She saw the need for a facility, and she created one. Today, the BFC is a model facility, an example and inspiration for other centers being created. Initiators of BFC have been asked, and responded, to help launch other residential rehabilitation programs.

Sometimes a graduate is so happy and impressed with the total life changes experienced by themselves and their families (who participate at BFC too), that they may have repeated Betty Ford's process and opened another center. Through recovery they developed a vision of a healthy community, where love and caring and connection could become a reality.

This phenomenon is happening over and over again. People who recover—whether it be at BFC or its equivalent, Daytop, Delancey Street, Merritt Peralta Institute, or any other place— want to share their experiences and help others do it. If you want help, or want to offer help to others, the possibility of making it happen materializes.

Like the Mimi Silberts, the Betty Fords, and the Monsignor O'Briens, there are many who will get together with like-minded friends and create a reality to fill a need. Any successful happening starts with a seed, a dream, or vision. And the rest falls into place when individuals are willing to share and cooperate. It is hard work and dedication, with disappointments along the way. But when you learn about these successful projects, you also learn that every minute of it was worth it to those who made it happen.

Information on how to contact these and other similar programs may be found in "Sources of Help" at the back of this book.

Endnotes to Chapter 7

1. These suggestions address the general population, recognizing that occasionally (one in several million)one experiences a spontaneous or "miracle" healing, usually as a result of a religious experience.

2. The Veterans Administration Hospital in La Jolla, California, conducted a study that showed that regular yoga and meditation increased blood levels of three important immune-system hormones by 100 percent. Many studies document that regular practice normalizes or lowers blood pressure and pulse rate. It produces changes in brain-wave patterns, showing less excitability, which in turn reflects changes in attitude. Meditation raises the pain threshold and reduces one's biological age.

3. Writing in *Family Therapy Networker* (July/August 1987), in an article entitled "Alcoholics Anonymous: From Surrender to Transformation," David Berensen states that the addict's task is to ". . . stop attempting to control by exerting willpower and open up to the discovery of a Higher Power. An alcoholic has to give up willfulness in favor of willingness . . . AA is perhaps unique among organizations in our culture in that it has been able to tap into the human thirst for oneness and belonging, while respecting individual dignity and avoiding coercive tactics, exploiting its members, or relying upon external support."

4. Hight, Jim, "New Uses for Acupuncture," IN *Yoga Journal* (January/February 1990), page 14. The Lincoln Hospital in the Bronx has been treating heroin addicts with acupuncture since the early 1970s. Today some 250 crack, heroin, and other drug addicts are treated daily. Janice O'Neil, drug counselor for 20 years, says acupuncture is the most effective method for drug detox that she has ever seen, offering immediate relief.

5. Temko, Allan, "Italian Look for Delancey Street Complex," IN *San Francisco Chronicle* (December 28, 1989).

6. Ibid.

7. From Pogash, Carol, "The Lady of the House—Mimi Silbert Inherits the Delancey Street Empire." Cover story in the Sunday *San Francisco Chronicle and Examiner, Image* magazine (July 31, 1989).

CHAPTER 8

Nutritional Therapies

Ongoing nutritional support is often critical in order to achieve a real and lasting recovery from addiction—and this fact is increasingly being recognized. Many of those who stay drug or alcohol-free merely substitute their chosen substance with large-scale use of coffee, sugar, and cigarettes. This indicates that the metabolic disorder underlying the addiction still exists and that the addict-prone are just transferring to other, more socially acceptable, addictive drugs.

Basic nutritional and metabolic disorders must be identified and corrected in order for a recovery program to have a long-term effect. This means providing people with a nutritional program that will help heal them, not only in the treatment facility, but after they leave.

The main requirements of this nutritional program are:

It must be effective.

It must be practical and easy to implement.

It must be relatively inexpensive.

The cornerstones of nutritional support are formulas that strengthen metabolism, increase energy, and heighten one's sense of well-being. Many of my clients who successfully broke free of alcohol, caffeine, sugar, and drug addictions have told me that within a matter of days or weeks of stopping their nutritional program, they began experiencing fatigue, irritability, depression, and insufficient energy to work competently. Simultaneously, they began getting strong cravings for their favorite substances for relief. As soon as they renewed the use of their nutritional formulas and good diet, they began feeling better and lost their cravings.

There is an enormous amount of medical literature showing the relationship of low thyroid function, weak adrenals, low levels of prostaglandins and nutritional deficiencies to cravings for addictive substances. In one experiment, healthy animals were put into cages with bowls of alcohol and bowls of water. As long as they were healthy, the animals didn't touch the alcohol. When their glands became stressed out or when a purposely-created nutritional deficiency existed in the animals, they chose alcohol over water. As soon as their nutrients or glandular strength was restored, the animals again avoided the alcohol. These tests have been repeated again and again with the same results.

In a recent study of patients receiving inpatient treatment for alcoholism, half received only the regular treatment plan and half received a nutritional program as well. Six months after discharge, only 33 percent of the patients in the regular program remained sober, whereas 81 percent of the nutritionally supported group remained sober.[1]

People who have been addicts or alcoholics for a period of time usually have developed severe glandular weakness and nutritional deficiencies. It takes at least several months to regenerate their glands and build their nutritional reserves. During this time, they need strong nutritional and metabolic support. Every few hours, their bodies will experience extreme biochemical disorders as their blood sugar drops, calcium, magnesium and zinc levels go out of whack, and their endocrine glands fail to produce adequate amounts of hormones. These biological disorders can create such pressures on their mental and emotional state that they feel severe depression and fatigue and are compulsively driven to utilize sugar, caffeine, nicotine, alcohol, and drugs for relief.

Replacement therapy is one of the main principles of this program. Stopping the drinking, drug-taking, and coffee and sugar use does not cure the metabolic disorder that causes depression, alienation, irritability, or fatigue. The answer is a nutritional formula that helps heal the disorder. It makes an enormous difference when a person trying to quit has a replacement formula that provides the nutrients his body lacks and gives strong metabolic support to his weakened glands and blood sugar mechanisms.

One of the best features of this program is that it is simple and inexpensive enough for people to put together and follow with the help of their physician. It is important to work with a nutritionally oriented physician where possible, because the possibilities of low thyroid, yeast overgrowth, and other disorders all need to be thoroughly checked.

FORMULAS FOR RECOVERY

The following formulas have proven to be effective in programs for recovering addicts and alcoholics, as well as for strengthening co-dependents who have weakened their health.

Concentrate Foods
Nutritional Yeast
Miso
Bee Pollen

Whole Food Extracts
Oils and Fats: Essential Fatty Acids
Flax Seed Oil
Omega Plus
Barley Green Extract
Fresh Carrot, Celery, Beet Juice
PC 55

Whole Food Herbs and Medicinal Herbs and Formulas
Liv. 52
Milk Thistle
Gamma Linolenic Acid

Korean Ginseng
Siberian Ginseng
Calendula (Marigold)
Calli Tea
Fortune Delight Tea
Prime Again
Beauty Pearls
Action Caps
NuPlus
Lifestream
Alpha 20C
Quinary
Top
Ese
Vitataste
Stevia
Goldenseal
Swedish Bitters
Dandelion Root
Km
Ginkgo Biloba
Chamomile
Peppermint
Scullcap

Minerals

Mezotrace
Multi Mineral (Whole Food Extract or good quality
    mineral chelate)
Zinc Picolinate
Calcium
Magnesium
Iron
Trace Minerals (Molybdenum, Manganese, etc.)
Potassium
GTF Chromium
Selenium

Amino Acids
  DL-Phenylalanine (DLPA)
  Glutamine

Vitamins
  Vitamin C
  Vitamin B Complex
  Vitamin E
  Vitamin A

Beneficial Digestive Floras
  Bifidus
  Acidophilus
  Streptococcus faecium

Enzymes
  S.O.D.

CONCENTRATED FOODS

Nutritional Yeast

Nutritional Yeast is an excellent food to use for those who are not allergic to it. It has a long established tradition of being very helpful in cases of fatigue, liver damage and hypoglycemia. It provides high amounts of all the B vitamins, protein, potassium, zinc, GTF chromium, RNA and other key nutrients. It can be added to soups or smoothies and sprinkled over popcorn. Many people mix yeast in a cup of miso broth for a quick pick-me-up. There are many different types of food yeast with widely varying tastes and nutritional contents. Some are the by-product of the brewing industry. The yeasts with the best taste and highest nutritional content are the primary grown: they are four to five times more nutritious than brewing industry byproducts, and they taste a lot better. Kal and Lewis Labs make excellent yeast flakes.

Miso

Miso is made from fermented soybeans which are usually combined with barley or other grain. It is a delicious addition to soups and salad dressings, providing easily digested complete protein. Unpasteurized miso is acclaimed for its ability to aid in digestion and assimilation of other foods. Miso comes in a variety of flavors, which vary in salt content, and bring out the flavor and nutritional value in foods. The oils contained in miso give it its savory flavor and aroma, and aid in dispersing accumulations of cholesterol and other fatty acids in the circulatory system. A major study conducted in Japan found that those who drank miso soup every day had 32 to 33 percent less stomach cancer than those who did not. In Japan, it is believed that miso promotes long life and good health, can cure colds, improve metabolism, clear the skin, and help resist parasitic diseases. It is also used to settle an upset stomach and get rid of a hangover. Miso has been found to contain dipicolinic acid, which attaches to radioactive metals and discharges them from the body. Some people have found that taking miso soup every day helps to alleviate the side effects of radiation therapy. It has also been found to neutralize the effects of smoking and air pollution.[2]

Bee Pollen

Bee pollen is one of mankind's oldest and most widely used nutritional and rejuvenating formulas. It is the only food that has all the proteins, vitamins, minerals, fats, and carbohydrates necessary to sustain life. It has also been found to contain special nutrients that strengthen the metabolism, endocrine glandular, and immune system functions. A large number of medical studies have been done showing its efficacy for fatigue, weakness, allergies, colds, neurasthenia, prostatitis, arthritis, and general degenerative conditions.

Each individual pollen granule is contained within a hard shell that resists digestion. Two companies (High Desert Pollen and 3rd Day Botanicals) have developed methods to fracture the hard exterior shell and make the vital inner nutrients available. A small percentage of people are allergic to pollen, but most can use it safely.

WHOLE FOOD HERBS AND MEDICINAL HERBS AND FORMULAS

Many research studies have shown that most diets are deficient in minerals, enzymes, vitamins, and other key nutrients, and that this is a major cause of health problems today.[3] One way to correct these deficiencies, or just to increase overall health and performance, is to include whole food concentrates in the daily diet.

No synthetically produced formula of vitamins, minerals, proteins, etc., has been made that will sustain human or animal life. Because science once thought that vitamins and minerals were completely separated from their whole food complexes before the body absorbed them, these manufactured chemicals were believed to be as valuable as the nutrition in foods. Recent groundbreaking research has shown that this is not the case.

A scientific study involving several laboratories and done over a period of two decades has revealed some startling new information that invalidated some existing beliefs regarding nutrient absorption and utilization in humans. The results of the study, which was headed by Siamak A. Adibi M.D., Ph.D. at the University of Pittsburgh School of Medicine, and supported by a grant from the National Institute of Arthritis, Metabolism, and Digestive Diseases, stunned the scientific community. Contrary to existing dogma that the intestine breaks down food nutrients to their isolated free-form molecular level, the newest evidence showed that the intestine breaks down food nutrients to the peptide complex level. This means food is broken down in the human body only to a level in which it is still molecularly bound to protein complexes and most likely carbohydrate, lipid, and bioflavonoid complexes as well. It is then absorbed into the bloodstream in complex peptide forms, identified by the appropriate cells, and utilized.

The research highlights critical differences between how food-extract nutrients and synthetic nutrients affect the body. Synthetic vitamins, which have little in common with nutrients found in foods and are in many cases entirely different chemical structures, can be useless to people with severely depleted liver function and an inability to absorb nutrients. For people with such damage, large doses of synthetic vitamins can actually be toxic and can cause severe damage to the liver, intestinal tract, kidneys, and nervous system. Food-grown minerals and food-complexed vitamins are highly assimilable by the body because they are grown on whole, living foods which "absorb" the vitamin or mineral they are "fed" and build a protein complex around them. These vitamin and mineral complexes are virtually identical to those found in food. They are highly assimilable and up to 1000 times more potent than the synthetic counterpart. Studies have shown that food-grown minerals and food-complexed vitamins exhibit far less toxicity than their synthetic counterparts, and are far better absorbed and retained than any others available.

About 12 years ago, an east coast company, Grow Company, Inc., successfully developed a proprietary process for "re-naturing" vitamin and mineral supplemental material. Food-grown supplements are now available through Grow Company's licensees: Rainbow Light, Mega Food, Lifestar, etc. As of this date, a total of 48 scientific studies have been completed, eight articles and 10 technical papers published, and six seminars presented at major Universities in Europe, documenting the differences between ordinary "natural" vitamins (USP) and "re-natured" protein-bound vitamins.

Organically-raised whole foods and whole food concentrates are an even better source of assimilable nutrients, except when people need higher amounts than can be found in foods and their concentrates. The best way to create a strong, healthy body and mind is to think and live well, eat wholesome foods supplemented by special herbal and whole food extracts and concentrates, and add careful use of good quality vitamin and mineral formulations to give that extra support.

WHOLE FOOD EXTRACTS

Essential Fatty Acids

While the realization is widespread that our foods and diets have become seriously deficient in key minerals, vitamins, fiber, amino acids, and often complex carbohydrates, it is only recently coming into general understanding that modern processing methods of fats and oils have created an even more serious problem of damage from poisonous, rancid oils and trans fatty acids, as well as serious deficiencies of Omega 3 and Omega 6 fatty acids and key prostaglandins.

The key to understanding the fats, oils, and cholesterol controversy is balance. The body requires cholesterol and the essential Omega 3 and Omega 6 fatty acids. It needs an entire range of minerals, proteins, and vitamins, and adequate levels of hormones. When any of these ingredients is too high or too low, disorder and disease will result.

Just as we need good quality protein, carbohydrate, vitamins and minerals, we need good quality fats and oils for physical and mental health. There are two types of fats, saturated and unsaturated. The saturated fats, found in butter, eggs, fish, chicken and meats, are high in cholesterol. The unsaturated fats are found in vegetable oils, such as sunflower, sesame, safflower, corn, and flax seed, and are high in the essential Omega 6 and Omega 3 fatty acids. The non-essential monosaturated fatty acids are found in olive and other oils.

We need a certain amount of both saturated and unsaturated fats in our diets. Except for people who have serious heart disease from a lifetime of poor eating and little exercise, most of us need a minimal amount of cholesterol in our diet. Over eight percent of our brain's solid matter is made of cholesterol; our hormones, skin, and even the membranes of our cells use cholesterol as an essential building block in their basic production and structure.[4, 5]

We also need the unsaturated fats—the Omega 6 and Omega 3 fatty acids found in the vegetable oils. It isn't a question of either/or—should I use saturated or unsaturated fats? Most of us need both in good quality forms. What we don't need are the refined or hydrogenated fats found in margarines, vegetable shortenings, or refined vegetable oils. Excellent information has been brought forth in recent years by Dr. Johanna Budwig, Dr. Ronald Rudin, Ann Louise Gittleman, Charles Bates, and others showing the critical need for the Omega 6 and Omega 3 fatty acids in our diets. These fatty acids provide our bodies with the raw materials to build the vital prostaglandins which, in many ways, are crucial to the recovering addict and alcoholic.[6] They are also good sources of energy, they are an essential part of the body's oxygen transport mechanism, and they are key building blocks of our skin, hormones, etc. Most of us obtain ample amounts of the Omega 6 fatty acids from safflower, sesame, sunflower, soy, canola, and corn oils, but we are seriously deficient in the Omega 3 fatty acids. The correct ratio of dietary Omega 6 and Omega 3 fatty acids should be 9 to 1, but modern diets often have an imbalance as severe as 12 to 1 Omega 6 to Omega 3 fatty acids. A deficiency of Omega 3's has been strongly implicated as a main cause of heart disease, cancer, immune system breakdown and other modern maladies. The only really concentrated sources of the Omega 3 fatty acid are flax seed oil and certain fish, such as mackerel, sardines, tuna, trout, and cold water salmon. This is why we need one or both of these in our diets.

To receive an adequate amount of both the Omega 6 and Omega 3 essential fatty acids, one should consume one to two tablespoons a day of high quality expeller pressed sesame, safflower or corn oil, and one to three teaspoons a day of expeller pressed flax seed oil.

Many people believe that because they buy their oils in a health food store with colorful labels featuring drawings of vegetables and statements like "expeller pressed" or "cold pressed" they are getting good quality oils. This is not the case.

The problems with most of the oils sold in health food stores and supermarkets are twofold: First, the vital nutrients (i.e., Omega 3 and Omega 6 fatty acids, vitamin E, lecithin, and beta carotene) are removed or destroyed. Second, there are serious poisonous substances created: trans fatty acids, free radicals, and peroxides.

Refined oils are subjected to several processing methods—deodorization, winterizing, bleaching, and alkali refining.[7, 8, 9] These processes remove virtually all the vitamin E, lecithin, and beta carotene.[10] Even worse, refining destroys the essential Omega 3 and Omega 6 fatty acids, converting them into poisonous trans fatty acids.[11, 12] The oils also develop a certain amount of rancidity, because they are processed in the presence of light and oxygen, then bottled in clear glass containers, which allow the light to penetrate and further their rancid deterioration.[13, 14] Light causes serious free radical damage to oils and light oxidation is 1000 times faster than oxygen oxidation.[15]

The deodorizing phase of the refining process is the worst. The oil is heated to a temperature of 470 degrees F., which removes the strong taste of the seed from which it is extracted.[16] Why do all these companies make such a big deal about their oils being extracted in a low temperature (which even at 140 to 160 degrees F. is still high enough to cause some damage and ideally should be extracted at temperatures below 118 degrees F.), and not inform us that they also subject the oils to a 470 degree temperature in the deodorizing process?

To insure that we do not burden our bodies with toxic substances and that we receive adequate intake of our essential fatty acids, we should use only high quality oils with extra flax seed oil or fish oil extracts, or include regular amounts of cold water fatty fish in our diets.

High quality oils need to be expeller pressed at temperatures below 118 degrees F. instead of solvent extracted. They should not be subjected to high heat temperatures, to deodorizing, bleaching, alkali refining, or winterizing processes. They need to be produced by light and oxygen excluded methods, bottled in containers that prevent the further exposure to light causing rancidity, and where possible they should be produced from organically grown seed.

At this time, there are only three companies producing oils meeting these standards of quality: Flora Oils, Galaxy Enterprises, Ltd., and Omega Nutrition in Canada, and Flora, Omega

Nutrition, and Arrowhead Mills, Inc./Omegaflo in the United States. Omega Nutrition, and Arrowhead Mills, Inc./Omegaflo, have the added advantage that the oils are bottled in completely light-excluding containers, and they are made exclusively from certified organically grown seed.

Flax Seed Oil

Next to oxygen, the nutrients used in the largest amounts in the body's metabolic processes are the Omega 6 and Omega 3 fatty acids. Absolutely necessary for health, we must obtain both essential fatty acids from what we eat.

Studies have found that one of the foremost nutritional deficiencies we are all subject to is that of the key Omega 3 fatty acid. An inadequate intake of this vital nutrient has been clearly linked with helping cause most modern diseases. Today, because of food processing the average diet contains only one-sixth of what we need and what the average diet in 1820 contained. Many doctors have found that alcoholics and addicts have deficiencies of these key fatty acids and that adding them to their program greatly aided recovery.[17, 18, 19]

The body uses the Omega 6 and Omega 3 fatty acids to produce energy and heat; to build strong cellular membranes that are resistant to pathogenic yeast, bacteria's, and viruses; to absorb and transport oxygen across the lung membranes into the bloodstream and into the cells; and to produce the essential prostaglandins that regulate immune system, glandular and nervous system functioning. These are just a few of the key functions of these fats.[20, 21, 22]

There are only two major sources of Omega 3: fish oils and flax seed oil. Flax seed oil is the richer source of Omega 3, requires less processing, tastes better, contains no toxic substances, is more stable, is less expensive, is a good source of the Omega 6 fatty acids, and has no cholesterol. Recommended daily usage is one to three teaspoons. It is a good tasting oil and can be poured directly on protein dishes, vegetables, salads, grains, soups, etc. It is a very delicate oil and should not be used for cooking.

The best flax seed oil is produced by Omega Nutrition, Arrow-head Mills/OmegaFlo, Galaxy Enterprises, and Flora.[23] It is extracted by all four companies from certified organically grown seed by a specially developed low-heat, oxygen-excluded method and the Omega Nutrition and Arrowhead Mills/OmegaFlo oils are bottled in light-insulated plastic containers.

Omega Plus

Omega Plus is a unique formula containing both flax seed oil and GLA from borage seed oil. This unique formulation is the only complete fatty acid formula that contains good amounts of both the essential Omega 3 and Omega 6 fatty acids, as well as GLA and the Omega 9 fatty acid. It is produced wholly from certified organic flax seed and borage seed grown without the use of herbicides and pesticides. Borage seed is a superior source of GLA, containing more than twice as much as evening primrose oil. The oils are expeller pressed at temperatures below 118 degrees F., in a light and oxygen excluding environment and bottled in light excluding containers.

Recommended usage is 2 to 3 capsules, 3 times daily.

Ingredients: Certified organic flax seed oil, borage seed oil.

Available in the United States from Leading Edge Nutrition and in Canada from SISU.

Barley Green Extract

This excellent product is the extract and concentrate of the juice of young green barley grass. It is a tremendous source of vitamins, minerals, proteins, and enzymes. It is seven times richer in Vitamin C than oranges, five times richer in iron than spinach, has nearly 11 times the calcium as milk, six times as much carotene as spinach and 30 times as much Vitamin B1 as milk. It is a tremendous alkalizer of the system, and one of the best foods to regenerate a damaged liver.

Fresh Carrot, Celery, and Beet Juice

Fresh carrot, celery, and beet juices are some of the best foods to heal the liver and build up the blood. These juices are full of highly assimilable vitamins, minerals, and enzymes, and are excellent cleansers as well as builders of health. These juices also improve adrenal and immune system function. Because of the high carbohydrate content, people with severe hypoglycemia and/or yeast overgrowth need to avoid them until they are stronger.

Recommended use is 8 to 12 ounces daily, preferably from organically-raised, pesticide-free vegetables. A good proportion is 60 percent carrot, 30 percent celery and 10 percent beet. A little parsley can also be added. Beet juice is a powerful liver cleanser and can cause a reaction in some people; therefore, it should be used carefully. It is very important to drink plenty of water and to dilute the juice 50 percent with water for those with blood sugar malfunction.

PC55

PC 55 is an extract and concentrate of the most powerful constituents of Lecithin. It has an important role to play in rebuilding the liver, nervous system, and cellular membranes. In Europe, doctors have used it successfully in treating hepatitis.[24, 25, 26, 27]

WHOLE FOOD HERBAL EXTRACTS

Herbal Formulas

Herbal formulas made with special extraction and concentration methods are among the most powerful substances known to regenerate and heal weak, deficient body systems.

Today's medical researchers are finding that elements like organic germanium,[28] Coenzyme Q10,[29] hormonal precursors, and tissue nutrients are some of the remarkable substances in these formulas that give them seemingly magical properties.

However, there are certainly yet-to-be discovered factors in them, and no isolated individual substances have been found that can duplicate the powerful effects of these concentrated nutrients for rebuilding and balancing disturbed body functions.

Some schools of natural healing believe most illnesses are caused by weakness of a particular glandular or organ system. The human body is composed of seven basic functioning systems: the digestive, nervous, glandular, respiratory, muscular, skeletal, and circulatory lymphatic systems. When illness manifests, rather than identifying and labeling tens of thousands of separate symptomatic disease entities and treating them as isolated events, we see that illness is often caused by weakness or imbalance of a total body system. We can then feel the person the foods and nutrients that will strengthen and regenerate the malfunctioning system and the disorder will clear up automatically.

This particular viewpoint of understanding and healing illness by strengthening the gland or organ system which governs it is gaining more and more acceptance today. This is due in part to the repercussions of many modern therapies: both the public and medical profession are witnessing the damaging side effects that are often a consequence of symptomatic treatment of disease.

Ivan Illich, in *Medical Nemesis,* and many other authoritative researchers, have repeatedly demonstrated the ineffectiveness of symptomatic treatment. More and more physicians today are turning to holistic methods of healing and some have taken an approach similar to that of the ancient sages—treating disease by feeding and strengthening different glands and organ systems. This may be seen in the works of Henry Bieler, M.D. in *Food is Your Best Medicine,* William McGarvey, M.D. in *The Edgar Cayce Remedies,* and Elliot Abravanel, M.D. in *Dr. Abravanel's Body Type Diet.*

There are three basic categories of plants: poisonous herbs; medicinal herbs to be used for temporary relief in emergency situations (these have dangerous side effects and must be used carefully); and, whole food herbs which supply nutrients that feed the glands and organs and help them to regenerate.

For instance, carrots and beets are whole food herbs that feed and help heal the liver; cabbage is a whole food herb that feeds and helps to heal the digestive tract. It must be emphasized that whole food herbal formulas are made from vegetables like carrots and cabbage and so are perfectly safe to use. They work by nourishing the body itself.

Following are some of the most potent herbs and herbal formulas. The best of them are grown using organic methods in very fertile soils which provide the plants with an abundance of nutrients and the proper humus conditions for the roots to assimilate them. They are picked at a specific time during growth when the healing properties are at the greatest potency. They are then mixed according to special formulas.

A primary factor in what makes formulations uniquely effective is the specialized extraction process developed for each herb. Many of the nutrients in herbs are bound up in the cellulose, in the complex protein molecules, and in other molecular combinations (fats, minerals) within the herbs. It is through highly complex and specific extraction techniques that the nutrients are separated from their bindings with other substances and made highly assimilable, even by weak and malfunctioning digestive systems.

All the ways in which these herbs and formulas help to regenerate the body will probably never be understood, but five principal functions are known. They provide: 1) essential nutrients in a concentrated, synergistically combined, highly assimilable form; 2) hormonal precursors; 3) adaptogens and enzymes; 4) antiviral, antibacterial, antifungal and antiparasitic properties; and 5) cleansing.

Most people do not drink enough cleansing fluids. The amount of water and teas needed varies greatly from individual to individual. Most people need at least 4 to 6 cups and some 12 to 16 cups daily. One should avoid following rigid programs and try to become more and more in touch with one's natural thirsts and appetites. One difficulty is that a body that has been abused and malnourished often loses its clear perception of what to eat and drink and often needs general guidance in the beginning.

Generally speaking the larger and more active the person and the warmer the climate, the more fluids a person needs to drink. Also, heavy meat and fat eaters need more fluids than those who eat moderately or who are semi or strict vegetarians.

When it comes to herb teas, while many of the commonly used beverage teas such as mint, chamomille, and others are generally beneficial for all to use, there are great differences in what herbs are best suited for use by each individual. One man's medicine is another man's poison certainly applies to the herbal kingdom. When working with imbalanced, ill, or recovering bodies, one needs to exercise great caution and wisdom in using medicinal herbs, as a powerful medicinal herb that is used injudiciously can cause real damage.

For those who find it is too much trouble to locate, blend, and prepare fresh teas, they can use the freeze dried extracts and concentrates with excellent results as well.

Herb teas come in six classes: fresh herbs, dried herbs, powdered extracts and concentrates, liquid extracts, tinctures, and powdered whole herbs that are tableted or encapsulated.

Generally the most potent are either the freshly brewed from fresh or dried whole herbs or the properly prepared freeze dried extracts and concentrates made by Sunrider, Himalaya Drug Co., Green Magma, Yerba Prima, Jarrow Formulas, and other companies. For the most part, the Chinese extracts and concentrates are much stronger than individual herbal teas.

Liquid extracts properly prepared and alcohol tinctures can have good value although many people, especially recovering addicts, have trouble with the alcohol tinctures. Bio Botannica has recently developed a line of alcohol-free herbal extracts, and people are trying them now to assess their effectiveness.

For the most part, the tablets and capsules composed simply of ground herbs are not anywhere as potent and effective as the freshly brewed teas or the quality extracts and concentrates.

When a tea is freshly prepared from fresh, preferably organically grown or wildcrafted herbs, the nutrients are extracted and put into a solution that is easily assimilated by the body and incorporated into its blood, tissue fluids, and cellular compositions.

This is especially important for people recovering from addictions and illness, as their digestive and assimilative capacities are often seriously compromised.

There is also a great difference in the cleansing and healing properties of herbs depending on whether they were organically grown or wildcrafted on fertile soils, gathered at the right time of year, the species of plant, dried and stored properly and on how old they are.

The packaged teas in bags offered by Celestial Seasonings and other companies are pleasant beverages and a welcome change from caffeine beverages; however, they have little therapeutic value because of the poor quality of the herbs and loss of properties incurred from processing, powdering and storage. Among the best of the companies making herb tea bags is Satori, who has come out with a line of exceptional quality herbal teas in tea bag form, including 8 single organic herbs in tea bags.

Liv.52

In the 1950s, the Himalaya Drug Company began a program screening more than 300 drugs and compounds to determine if, histopathologically, they could help in the protection or regeneration of the hepatic parenchyma while other tests were used to measure improvement in liver function. (Despite the advances of modern medical research, no drug was available to help the liver to regenerate after damage, stimulate liver function, and protect it.) All drugs or compounds found useful were scrupulously checked for their chronic and acute toxicity since treatment of the diseased liver is necessarily prolonged.[30]

Of all the drugs and compounds screened and tested, the compound bearing the code number "Liv.52" showed extreme promise. This was then given for clinical trials and soon a number of papers were published on the efficacy of Liv.52.

Over three decades of extensive controlled laboratory studies, clinical trials, and medical usage has shown Liv.52 to be remarkably safe, non-toxic, and free from side effects. In fact, no LD 50 (lethal dose at which 50 percent of laboratory animals die when administered a pharmaceutical compound) has ever been established. In other words, there is no toxicity level. Experimental animals simply gain weight on Liv.52.

The following claims made for Liv.52 are supported by tissue culture studies, electron microscopy, radio isotope studies, biochemical assays, histopathological studies, and animal experiments.[31]

Liv.52 has been used successfully to treat a wide variety of severe liver disorders including:
• Viral hepatitis A and B
• Chronic hepatitis
• Alcoholic cirrhosis and pre-cirrhotic conditions
• Jaundice
• Infantile liver disorders.

This is critically important because modern medicine has no specific treatments for these most prevalent causes of liver disease.

Liv.52 has also been used successfully to treat liver disease resulting from administration of prescription drugs, such as corticosteroids, barbituates, anticancer agents, antibiotics, antitubercular drugs, and oral contraceptives. Liv.52 also protects against liver damage due to common analgesics such as acetaminophen.[32]

Liv.52 has been used prophylactically against liver damage due to exposure to alcohol, and hepatotoxic drugs and chemicals; against liver damage due to drugs including antibiotics, and to protect children with a family history of liver disease.[33]

Liv.52 has also been successfully used with the following conditions: to speed wound healing in severely burned patients; treat anorexia associated with chemotherapy; in the treatment of toxemia of pregnancy; speeding the recovery of malnourished children.[34]

Liv.52 has marked anabolic action, speeding recovery after illness and reducing convalescence after debilitating disease. It also encourages growth and improves a sense of well-being in underweight patients.

In experimental animals Liv.52 offers profound protection against radiation sickness. It counteracts hepatotoxic agents, including solvents and metals such as cadmium and beryllium.[35]

Liv.52 is a powerful hepatic stimulant. Typical results range from normalization of liver function tests to regeneration of liver parenchyma. It promotes hepatic cellular metabolism (increased glycogen deposition and increased bilirubin production), increases the production of serum proteins, and lowers elevated serum lipids.[36]

Liv.52 has been used extensively for the past 30 years. Millions of patients have used Liv.52 in India. Billions of doses have been administered. More than 4.5 billion tablets have been exported. Liv.52 has achieved drug status in Switzerland, U.S.S.R., and India. Total annual sales of Liv.52 approach 25 million bottles.

Dosage: 2 to 3 tablets, 3 times daily.

Liv.52 is much more than a carefully balanced formulation of herbomineral principles, useful in hepatic problems. It incorporates the essence of Ayurveda in a rational formulation designed to combat liver injury and to protect the liver against damage.

The Liv.52 formulation incorporates renowned Ayurvedic plant principles. For instance, Capparis spinosa is an appetite stimulant and reduces oedema. The quath (extracts) of the processed seeds of Chicorium intybus controls nausea and vomiting. Solanum nigrum and the leaves of Cassia occidentalis are mild laxatives (an action that is desirable in the early stages of hepatitis with bile stasis).

Each coated and imprinted Liv.52 tablet contains:

Capparis spinosa	65mg
Chichorium intybus	65mg
solanum nigrum	32mg
Cassia occidentalis	16mg
Terminalia arjuna	32mg
Achillea millefolium	16mg
Tamarix gallica	16mg
Mandur bhasma	33mg

The formula is currently available from your local doctor or pharmacy via SISU.

Milk Thistle

Milk Thistle extracts have been shown to have remarkable protecting and healing effects in treating many liver diseases, including cirrhosis, chronic hepatitis, chemical and alcohol-induced fatty liver, and several other disorders. With the tremendous increase in liver disease today brought on by excessive use of alcohol and drugs, and from the increased intake of poisons from the environment and food, this humble plant is certain to become one of the most sought after cures offered to man.

Numerous scientific studies have shown it works in several ways, and has been used successfully to treat patients with hepatitis and cirrhosis.[37] Milk thistle is currently used in European pharmaceutical preparations for hepatic disorders.[38] It protects the liver cell membranes from damage by poisons. It also increases protein synthesis in the liver and promotes the regeneration of new liver cells.[39] Cirrhosis-induced rats treated with milk thistle showed an appreciable decrease in hepatic collagen.[40] Gerard, the famous English herbalist, wrote: "My opinion is that this is the best remedy that grows against all melancholy (liver) diseases."

There are many grades of quality in milk thistle extracts. Some authorities state that the complete extract of the seed is best, while others feel that the isolated silibum compound within the seed is the best to use. I usually have found that the complete extract of an herb is best to use rather than one isolated nutrient, as there are usually many compounds in an herb that are a part of its synergistic healing effect.

Some of the best whole milk thistle extracts in the United States are produced by Bio Botannica and Herb Pharm, which can be obtained from Threshold or your health food store. These extracts are in an alcohol tincture, however, and if you are sensitive to the alcohol, you can boil it off or else use the isolated compound instead. Of the isolated milk thistle silymarin compounds, Yerba Prima, Planetary Formulas, and Phyto Pharmica make excellent alcohol-free preparations. One can also buy the whole or broken seeds and make a most potent tea by simmering 1 to 2 teaspoons of seeds for each cup of water for an hour.

Gamma Linolenic Acid

Gamma linolenic acid, usually derived from borage seed or evening primrose oil, provides the necessary raw materials for the body to make some of its crucial prostaglandins. This has several important uses in the recovering alcoholic's program. First, it is felt that a deficiency in needed prostaglandins can be a main metabolic factor causing the mental-emotional depression and imbalance that often leads to a craving for addictive substances. Use of gamma linolenic acid will help correct this biochemical malfunction.

Second, preliminary tests in humans have shown that gamma linolenic acid can make withdrawal from alcohol easier and can relieve post-drinking depression.[41, 42]

Dr. John Rotrosen and Dr. David Sagarnick at New York University did similar tests on mice. They made mice addicted to alcohol by giving them an alcohol-rich diet. They then took away the alcohol abruptly. Over the next few hours there was a dramatic withdrawal syndrome, similar to what happens with human alcoholics. The doctors then injected PGEI into the animals. This dramatically alleviated the withdrawal problems in the addicted mice. Tremor, irritability, over-excitability, and convulsions were all reduced by about 50 percent.[43] Gamma linolenic acid had the same effect as PGEI in preventing withdrawal symptoms.

Third, gamma linolenic acid has shown significant effects in healing liver damage caused by alcohol abuse. A very recent study done at the Alcoholic Clinic at Craig Dunaine Hospital in Inverness showed that gamma linolenic acid can go a long way in correcting liver damage due to alcohol.

Under consultant psychiatrist Dr. Iain Glen, the clinic conducted a double-blind trial with about 100 patients. No one knew who was taking capsules of gamma linolenic acid and who was taking identical capsules containing liquid paraffin.

The group who took evening primrose oil as a source of gamma linolenic acid did much better than the others. The results showed that gamma linolenic acid can improve liver function, reduce the demand for tranquilizers, improve brain function, and lower the incidence of hallucinations during the period of alcohol withdrawal. The liver in particular seemed to benefit; its biochemistry returned to normal much more rapidly among the patients taking gamma linolenic acid.

Dr. Glen was working on the hypothesis that drinking can seriously alter the body's membrane lipids. When he delivered his paper to an International Conference on Pharmacological Treatments for Alcoholism in London in March 1983, he said: "We used evening primrose oil because it contains a large amount of gamma linolenic acid. These membrane changes can block the linolenic acid metabolism. So, by giving alcoholics capsules of Efamol (evening primrose oil), we hoped to bypass this trouble." Dr. Glen said that evening primrose oil is the first specific medicine to show promise in treating alcohol dependence.[44] Since then, researchers have discovered that borage seed oil has twice as much GLA as evening primrose oil. They have also found that giving people flax seed oil as well provides the body with the necessary precursors for it to make other important prostaglandins.[45]

In one of the most recent books to date on this subject, *Essential Fatty Acids and Immunity in Mental Health*, Charles Bates, Ph.D., describes the cases of many recovering alcoholics who were greatly aided by the use of gamma linolenic acid. He found that some people have an inability to convert Omega 6 fatty acids into the essential PGE1 and PGE2 prostaglandin series. This is further compounded by the fact that most people also have excessive amounts of poisonous trans fatty acids and serious deficiencies of the Omega 3 and PGE3 prostaglandin series. What Bates found is that the PGE1 and PGE2 prostaglandin deficiency causes chronic depression and fatigue, but that drinking alcohol caused a temporary increase in the release of prostaglandins which alleviated the depression and fatigue. This effect was only temporary—later the conditions worsened. Using gamma linolenic acid resulted in an increase in the manufacture of the PGE1 and PGE2 prostaglandin series, the depression and fatigue cleared up, and most of the craving for alcohol disappeared.

Korean White Ginseng

Ginseng is considered the king of tonic herbs. It feeds and strengthens the endocrine glands and overall metabolism. "The ginsenosides have immunomodulatory activity; they stimulate the biosynthesis of proteins in rat liver and kidney and increase plasma levels of ACTH and corticosterone. They control homeostasis by acting on the endocrine system."[46] Athletes use ginseng to increase their stamina and people recovering from addictions using ginseng to build their health. It is used to strengthen the heart and normalize blood pressure. It also nourishes the blood, having a beneficial effect on anemia.

Its use is especially indicated for those with weak adrenal or reproductive glandular function, and those with hypoglycemia, fatigue and nervous system weakness.

This herb has special catalyzing properties and will increase the effectiveness of other herbs when used with strengthening herbal formulas.

Three to 6 capsules a day is the recommended dosage.

Siberian Ginseng Root

This herb nourishes the spleen-liver function and helps strengthen joint tissues, ligaments, and tendons. Traditionally, it has been used for lack of appetite, insomnia, forgetfulness, nervous disorders, low energy, and convalescent weakness. A review of studies in which Siberian ginseng was given to over 2000 healthy human subjects found that it increased their ability to withstand adverse physical conditions, increased mental alertness and improved work production and athletic performance. In another review of clinical trials given to over 2000 human subjects with a variety of illnesses, it was found to aid healing of both low and high blood pressure, improve adrenal and thyroid function, help prevent some forms of cancer, help heal many other illnesses and increase overall sense of well-being. This information was reviewed from several research studies in an extract from the Townsend Letter in the January 1989 *Phyto-Pharmica Review*, Volume, 2, Number 1. Three to 6 capsules daily is the recommended dosage.

Calendula

Calendula (marigold flowers) makes an excellent, soothing tea that is healing to the digestive tract and liver. Its high content of allantoin promotes the growth of new cell tissues. European herbalists have used it for centuries as an aid to healing hepatitis, both A and B types. It also has powerful antifungal and antibacterial properties that make it an excellent preventative and therapeutic remedy for yeast overgrowth. For disorders of the liver or yeast overgrowth, one should drink 3 to 4 cups daily. One can prepare tea from fresh or dried flowers or use extracts prepared by Bio Botannica. Prepare by bringing water to a boil and steeping 1 teaspoon per cup of water for 5 to 10 minutes.

Calli Tea

This is a very powerful deep tissue cleanser. It improves liver function, aids fat metabolism, increases energy, strengthens digestion, and improves nervous system function and mental clarity. This is a very pleasant tasting tea. Many people find that it is not only very beneficial to their health but enjoyable as well.

The best and most remarkable formula I have seen for helping to free people from caffeine addiction is Calli tea. I have been amazed by the number of people who have told me that as soon as they began drinking Calli, they lost all craving for caffeine and were able to completely quit coffee and cola addictions with ease. One older, heavy-set woman was dependent on four quarts of coffee a day for the energy she needed to work and support herself and her family. As soon as she began using Calli, she quit without even desiring coffee.

Many people get enhanced benefit from adding Fortune Delight tea to the Calli. This is especially beneficial for those who tend to be overweight and have a slow metabolism.

Begin by steeping one Calli tea bag in a quart of boiled water for five minutes. Then start with one half to one cup per day after mealtime. Use only during the day at first. Once you have developed a feeling for using this tea, experiment with concentration and amount.

Ingredients: Camellia leaf, Perilla Leaf, Mori Bark Extract, Alisma Root Extract, Imperate Root, and other herbs as flavoring.

Caution: People with large amounts of stored drug or toxic deposits, or the severely ill, should begin using the tea in very dilute amounts. It can cause strong cleansing reactions in some people.

Fortune Delight Tea

This formula cleanses the digestive tract, kills yeast, improves digestion, and aids fat and cholesterol metabolism. It nourishes the nervous system and increases energy and stamina. It is especially good as a kidney, bladder, and urinary tract cleanser. People often experience slight nausea and intestinal upset initially as it kills yeast colonies and cleans toxic matter from the digestive tract. Begin by mixing 1 teaspoon of powdered tea in a quart of water and drink 1 to 2 cups a day. Increase the concentration and amount as your system adjusts to it. (Many people use 1 to 3 quarts a day and find that it greatly enhances their sense of well-being.) This tea has similar cleansing properties to Calli tea and thus the same directions and cautions for use apply. Excessive discomfort can be mitigated by using a more dilute amount, mixing it with dilute Calli or taking it with food. (There is a small amount of caffeine in Calli and Fortune Delight teas, but not enough to bother most people. Most of the caffeine is extracted in the processing.)[47] The two teas can be mixed together to produce a beverage with much greater and more complete cleansing and metabolic effects.

Ingredients: Camellia extract, Lemon extract, Chrysanthemum flower extract, Jasmine extract, Lalang grass root extract, King fruit extract, and other herbs as flavoring.

Prime Again: Endocrine Glandular Formula

This preparation feeds and improves functions of the endocrine glands, including the adrenals, thyroid, and reproductive glands. These glands produce hormones which are essential to life and regulate all the body's major functions and energy cycles. Among these are blood sugar level, protein assimilation and muscle building, nervous system function, mental well-being, immune system function, detoxification of poisons, digestive processes, body stamina, body temperature, and other essential body processes.

Most people with serious addictions have weakened their adrenal function. Prime Again is one of the best formulas to help restore endocrine glandular capacity.

Many illnesses, from arthritis to a susceptibility to recurrent infectious diseases and many vague bodily disorders such as fatigue, overweight, poor digestion, and poor nervous system strength are caused by weak or under-functioning glands. Strengthening and improving the glands' functions often clears up a whole host of disorders and dramatically improves overall health and personal enjoyment of life. This has been well documented by many authoritative researchers including: Broda Barnes, M.D. in *Hypothyroidism: The Unsuspected Illness*; Stephen Langer, M.D., on *Solved: The Riddle of Illness*; J.W. Tintera, M.D. in *Hypoadrenocorticism*; and Ray Peat, Ph.D. in *Nutrition for Women*, among others.

Prime Again, as well as flax seed oil, Beauty Pearls, Korean Ginseng Extract, Calli tea, Action Caps, and NuPlus have all demonstrated safe, repeated success in feeding and improving function of the endocrine glands. Irregular menstruation, PMS and menopausal symptoms have been greatly helped when

Prime Again is taken along with flax seed oil, GLA, and Beauty Pearls. Recommended dosage is 3 to 6 capsules a day for mild to moderate conditions and up to 12 daily for severe conditions.

Ingredients: Radix Dioscoreae, Radix Cyathulae, Herba Epimedium, Semem Allium, Poria, Fructus Corni, Fructus Broussonetiae, Cortex Eucommiae., Fructus Schizandrae, Fadix Morindae, Herba Cistanches, Radix Polygalae, Fructus Foeniculi, Rhizoma Acori Graminei.

Beauty Pearls: Women's Glandular Formula

This formula strengthens the endocrine glandular system and nourishes and improves the growth and healing processes. It specifically feeds the female hormonal system and often has a remarkable effect on improving PMS and menopausal symptoms. It increases energy and helps calm and stabilize the nervous system.

Women often experience such severe PMS that they develop extreme cravings for chocolate, sugar, alcohol, and drugs, in order to raise their blood sugar and alleviate the pain and stress. Regular use of Beauty Pearls, combined with flax seed oil, GLA, Dong Quai, NuPlus, Prime Again, and a good diet has been repeatedly found to greatly improve this condition.

Many people find this formula to be very strengthening and healing. For maintenance purposes use 1 tablet daily with meals. For more therapeutic uses take 2 tablets daily. Beauty Pearls contains extract of real pearl, which has traditionally been revered in the Orient as a source of special elements that rejuvenate the body's vital processes.

Ingredients: Honey, Korean Ginseng, Chrysanthemum Flower Extract, Royal Jelly Extract, Pearl, and other herbs as flavoring.

Action Caps

A very powerful preparation with broad effects on many body functions. Excellent for weight management, it helps restore normal fat metabolism function. Many people report not only a loss of excess fat but a building of lean muscle tissue as well. It picks up stamina and overall body energy, is a superlative cleanser of the digestive tract, and also improves the spleen-pancreas, liver, digestive, and glandular functions, all important factors in healing addictions. This formula is also great for building muscle tissue and strength in those who are under-weight. Action Caps consist of three separate formulas, to be taken together 2 or 3 times daily in a dosage of 2 to 3 capsules of each according to individual need.

Ingredients: Chinese Yam, Taro Powder, Plantago Asiatic, Tora Seed Powder, Camellia Leaf Extract, Imperate Root Extract, Caulis Hocquartial Extract, Rhizoma Alismatis Extract, Brigham Tea Extract, Senna Seed Extract, Rehmannia Glutinosa Extract, Cortex Mori Radicus Extract, and other herbs as flavoring.

NuPlus

NuPlus is among the most powerful herbal rebuilding formulas known. It has a strong regenerating effect on the adrenals, reproductive glands, liver, pancreas, kidneys, and nervous system. It helps build lean muscle tissue, improves fat metabolism and greatly increases stamina and energy. Athletes use it in large amounts to improve performance, and people convalescing from illness find it substantially aids their recovery.

People with severe fatigue or blood sugar problems and those recovering from addictions will find that it greatly stabilizes the metabolism and increases energy when used several times a day.

NuPlus mixes up best in a blender. Maintenance usage is 1 to 3 teaspoons once or twice a day. For building strength or recovering from an illness, use 2 to 3 teaspoons 3 times daily. Mix it in Calli tea and take it with Action Caps, Prime Again, Korean Ginseng, and Beauty Pearls.

Ingredients: Coix Fruit, Chinese Yam, Fox Nut, Lotus Seed, Lotus Root, Water Lily Bulb, and Imperate Root.

Lifestream: Circulatory System Formula

Improving circulation helps to alleviate depression and poor nervous system function and to cleanse poisons from the systems of those recovering from addiction. Poor circulation is a factor in many illnesses. A decreased blood supply to the brain and nervous system will cause depression and poor memory. A diminished blood supply to body tissues and organs will cause a decreased amount of oxygen and nutrients and a buildup of toxins, creating favorable conditions for all types of disease to develop.

This formula increases vascular elasticity and helps heal circulatory disorders, including varicose veins, hardening of the arteries, blood pressure malfunctions, excessive fat and cholesterol levels. It can also improve eyesight. Use 3 to 6 capsules daily for mild to moderate conditions and prevention of illness. Use up to 16 capsules per day for severe or chronic conditions.

Ingredients: Cassia Tora Seed, Gou Teng, Sophora Flower, Chrysanthemum Flower, Orange Peel, Pineliae Root, Dwarf Lilly, Turf Root, Poria (Mushroom Powder), Ginger Root, and Ginseng Root.

Alpha 20C

This formula is indicated for those who need to improve liver and immune system function. It has been very helpful for people with chronic Candida Albicans overgrowth and Epstein-Barr syndrome. Recommended dosage is 2 to 6 capsules daily. Up to 16 capsules daily is recommended for severe or chronic conditions. Very severe cases can use 25 to 50 capsules a day for a short duration to aid recovery.

Ingredients: Chinese White Flower, Paris Herb, Scutellaria Herb, Dandelion, and Imperate Root.

Quinary

This ancient and comprehensive formula was designed to nourish and strengthen the five major systems of the body. It provides key nutrients to the endocrine glandular, respiratory, circulatory, digestive, and liver-immune systems. This formula increases the strength and proper functioning of the entire body.

Addicts who have damaged their health should take it several times a day to build up their strength. Healthy people and athletes can take it, along with NuPlus, Calli, and Fortune Delight to stay strong and fit.

Ingredients: Chinese White Flower, Scutellaria Herb, Dandelion Root, Gou Teng, Licorice Root, Tora Seed, Mint Herb, Paris Herb, Orange Peel, Coix Fruit, Fennel Seed, Cinnamon Bark, Poria (Mushroom Powder), Chinese Yam, Ginger Root, Barren Wort Herb, Hawthorn Berry, Chuan Xiong Root, Mongoliavine Fruit, Golden Bell Fruit, Sophora Flower, Fung Fong Root, Ginseng Root, Honey Suckle Flower (Silver Flower), Yuan-Hu Root, Ostrea Shell, Chrysanthemum Flower, Dipsace Root, Angelica Root, Alpina Ginger Root, Angelica Centis Root, Leek Seed, Baloon Flower Root, Bamboo Leaf, Dwarf Lilly Turf Root, Paper Mulberry, Senega Root, Imperate Root, Connel Fruit, Forty-Knot Root, Burdock Fruit, Cnidium Fruit, Reed Root, Rhubarb Root, Broom Rape Herb, Chinese Catnip, Asias Herb, Bai-Zhu Root, Boxthorn Fruit, Eucommia Bark and Morinda Root.

Nervous System Formulas

Scientific research today is turning up evidence supporting what the Chinese sage doctors knew thousands of years ago. Recent studies on the health and functioning of the nervous system have discovered that certain key nutrients, neurotransmitters, prostaglandins, and hormones are essential to normal nervous system perception and function.

Stress, drug and alcohol abuse, poor nutrition, poisons, and genetic impairment can all contribute to creating a deficiency of these substances which will, in turn, cause serious malfunction of the nervous system.

The works of Dr. Fox in *DLPA*, Judy Graham in *Evening Primrose Oil*, Dr. Langer in *Solved: The Riddle of Illness*, and others have clearly shown the critical effect that these substances can have in clearing up depression, fatigue, and phobias, and in alleviating the pain of withdrawal, arthritis, and other diseases by strengthening nervous system function.

Today's pharmaceutical pain killers work by deadening the nervous system, and all have certain side effects. Proper use of nutrients and food herb formulas work by nourishing, normalizing, and increasing the capacity of the nervous system to function well under stress.

While there is clearly a place for using individual substances in improving nervous system function, the most important thing is to provide complete nourishment of all essential nutrients through the use of whole foods and whole food extracts.

The importance of calcium in maintaining normal nervous system functioning is well known, but what is not so well known is the difference in absorption and utilization of commonly used supplemental calcium products as opposed to calcium taken from whole foods.

Many scientific studies have shown that there is a great difference in the amount of calcium or any other nutrient the body is able to absorb and utilize, depending on whether it comes from food or food concentrates or from an isolated, synthesized nutrient.[48]

This is a major reason why foods and food extracts have such superior healing properties.

Since the endocrine glandular system (mainly the thyroid, adrenals, and reproductive glands) contributes at least 50 percent of the strength of the nervous system, the basic program should provide ample amounts of NuPlus, Flax Seed Oil, protein, Prime Again, and Beauty Pearls, along with Calli and Fortune Delight Teas.

Top

This formula is used with Ese (below) to enhance mental acuity. Some computer operators have reported that by using 2 to 3 capsules of Top and 2 capsules of Ese, they can work twice as long without mental fatigue. This formula is also good for headaches, neck and shoulder tension, insomnia, and mental difficulties.

People with allergies have reported that using Top, Ese, Alpha 20C, and Prime Again has cleared up their allergic conditions. Besides giving immediate relief, continued use over a period of time will help the body to heal the underlying disorder and aid permanent recovery. Dosage is 2 to 3 capsules once or twice daily, and more often during serious illness.

Ingredients: Mint, Silver Flower, Chuang-Xiong Root, Yeuan Wu Root, Angelicae Root, Golden Bell Fruit, Ji Tsau Herb, White Willow Bark.

Ese

This is the basic formula for strengthening nervous system function. Its use is indicated in conditions of general pain, burnout, and arthritis. It is used to aid mental concentration and clarity. Dosage is 2 to 3 capsules once or twice daily, and more often during serious illness.

Ingredients: Cassia Tora Seed, Gou Teng, Ji Tsau Herb, Sophora Flower, Yeuan Wu Root, Orange Peel, Pinelliae Root.

Vitataste

A healthy, well-nourished organism is physically satisfied and has no unnatural cravings for sugar or other stimulating, addictive substances. Sugar cravings can be caused by low endorphin levels, low endocrine hormones, nutritional deficiencies (especially B vitamins and zinc), low blood sugar, lack of exercise, and the yeast overgrowth syndrome. Effectively dealing with sugar cravings requires correcting the root causes and often needs a complete nutritional, glandular rejuvenating, and antiyeast overgrowth program.

One traditional Chinese herbal formula that corrects many of the nutritional and metabolic imbalances is Vitataste. This formula is very helpful, especially when used with a complete

program. Applying ⅛ of a capsule to the tongue causes chocolate, sugar, and other sweets to taste like sand. The effect lasts for
three hours. It also helps curb cravings for cigarettes and has
helped many to quit smoking altogether.

Ingredients: Lycii Fruit, Wuxue Teng, Coix Fruit, Lotus Seed,
Lotus Root, Water Lily Bulb, Imperate Root, Fox Nut.

Stevia

Stevia has a long history of safe and therapeutic use both as an
herbal sweetener and as an antifungal, anti-inflammatory and
antibiotic agent. It has been used for centuries by the natives in
South America and for the last few decades in Japan, where it is
much acclaimed by their medical professionals as a dentifrice
and a blood sugar stabilizer.

It is 30 times sweeter than sugar, yet has practically no sugar
in it. It has been found to lower the blood sugar in diabetics and
raise the blood sugar in hypoglycemics.

It is also remarkably efficacious when used topically for
poison oak, athletes foot, rashes, and infections.

Golden Seal

This herb is superior for cleansing the liver and bloodstream.
Golden seal was considered to be the finest blood purifier and
herbal antibiotic by such renowned authorities as Jethro Kloss,
Dr. John Christopher, and several others. People with liver
damage, infectious diseases, yeast disorders, and ulcerated
gastrointestinal tracts have found 3 to 6 capsules a day for 1 to 3
months to be of great aid in healing these conditions. More may
be taken during acute illness. Golden seal should not be taken for
more than three months nor used by pregnant women.

Swedish Bitters

This traditional formula, so popularized by Maria Treben in her
excellent book *Health Through God's Pharmacy*, is excellent for
stimulating appetite, improving liver function, and greatly aids

in healing and normalizing the digestion, glandular and nervous system functions. Take 1 teaspoon in 4 ounces of warm tea or water a half hour before and after each meal.

Dandelion

Dandelion root is considered to be one of the foremost herbs to improve liver function. It is used both as a food and a medicine. This herb increases the flow of bile and improves digestion, purifies the blood, and acts as a diuretic. It is considered to be one of the best remedies for blood toxicity, liver sluggishness or disorder, jaundice, hepatitis, gout, and arthritis.[49, 50]

Three to 6 capsules daily or prepare a fresh tea by bringing water to a boil and simmer 1 teaspoon dried root per cup of water for 30 to 60 minutes.

Km

This is a remarkable herbal extract and mineral formulation with powerful rejuvenating and cleansing properties. Many people have found it greatly increases their energy and stamina, cleanses poisons from the body, helps arthritis and other toxic conditions, helps rebuild the liver and the blood, and greatly increases the oxygenation of the system.

Its iodine and herbal content will improve thyroid function and strengthen the overall metabolic rate. This is especially important today, as many people suffer from subnormal thyroid function which can cause a pervasive weakening of their strength, health, and sense of well being. Regular intake of iodine supplementation is critical for everyone, as it protects the body against poisoning from radioactive fallout which is something we are all exposed to today, thanks to nuclear testing, Chernobyl, etc. The high level of potassium makes it very helpful for people with depleted adrenal function, those with nutritional deficiencies, and especially for people going through withdrawal and cleansing programs. Potassium deficiency is a widespread problem today. Excessive consumption of salt, use of caffeine, drugs, alcohol, and sugar, and poor dietary habits all contribute to the development of a potassium deficiency. Some pharmaceuticals like Cortisone, Prednisone, and diuretics can also create a potassium deficiency. This deficiency is a major cause of high blood pressure and heart disease, and many scientific studies have established that normalizing potassium intake results in normalizing blood pressure levels.[51] Low potassium levels also weaken adrenal and liver function.

Many report improved digestion and bowel regularity, relief from sensitive skin disorders, improvement of chronic respiratory weakness, and considerable reduction in musculo-skeletal pain and joint swelling when using this formula. Athletes say their energy levels are sustained for a longer period of time. Chronic urinary tract problems and other systemic difficulties also demonstrate improved levels of wellness.

For a maintenance dose, use 2 tablespoons a day. Km can initiate strong cleansing symptoms in people with large amounts of stored toxins. Those with serious toxicity or illness should begin with a small amount of Km, 1 tsp., and increase the dosage gradually until finding the amount that works best for them.

Ingredients: Potassium Citrate, Calcium Glycerophosphate, Potassium Glycerophosphate, Ferric Glycerophosphate, Chamomile Flowers, Sarsaparilla Root, Celery Seed, Angelica Root, Dandelion Root, Horehound Herb, Licorice Root, Senega Root, Passion Flower, Thyme, Gentian Root, Saw Palmetto Berry, Alfalfa, Cascara Sagrada, Potassium Hydroxide and Potassium Iodide.

Ginkgo Biloba

This exceptional herb is certain to be more and more in the news as time goes on. "Its actions include vasodilation, enhanced energy production, increased cellular glucose uptake, inhibition of platelet aggregation, free radical scavenging, and modulation of calcium flux. Its pharmacological activity is related to its high content of terpenes, flavonoids, proanthocyanidins, and ginkgo heterosides (flavoglycosides)."[52]

Many people in recovery suffer from depression, loss of memory, poor circulation, and failing eyesight. This herb has shown to increase cerebral blood flow as well as oxygen and glucose utilization, which help alleviate these conditions. It also has been found to be helpful in cases of vertigo, headache, and tinnitus. Use tablets or capsules as directed, or prepare fresh tea by bringing water to a boil and steeping 1 teaspoon per cup of water for 5 to 10 minutes.

Chamomile

This tea is an excellent herb for helping heal a damaged liver. Chamomile is one of a few plants that have been established to have properties which rebuild the liver. In a laboratory test, two compounds of chamomile (azulene and guaiazulene) were found to initiate new growth of liver tissue in rats which had portions of their livers surgically removed.[53]

Chamomile is also an excellent tea to use for relaxing the nervous system and for calming and strengthening the stomach. It has been found to neutralize twice as much stomach acid as the leading over-the-counter antacid. It also has powerful antifungal capabilities and is a good tea to use in cases of Candidiasis.[54, 55]

It has long been a favorite remedy for simple tension, nervousness, anxiety, insomnia, and upset stomach caused by excessive acidity. Prepare by bringing water to a boil and steeping 1 teaspoon per cup of water for 5 to 10 minutes.

Peppermint

Peppermint is one of the finest herbs for improving digestion and promoting liver function. It has a gently stimulating and refreshing influence on the nervous system. Its oils have strong antifungal, antibacterial, and antiviral activity.[56] It also has antiinflammatory and ulcer healing effects.[57] It is recommended to alleviate colds, indigestion, bilious, and headache conditions.

Prepare by bringing water to a boil and steeping 1 teaspoon per cup of water for 5 to 10 minutes.

Scullcap

For as long as history has been recorded, this herb has been used as one of the most reliable nervine tonics. It is considered one of the best herbs for breaking addictions and easing withdrawal symptoms and to have strong healing properties towards rebuilding depleted or burned out nervous systems.

"It has been clinically tested in China in patients with chronic hepatitis, where it improved symptoms in over 70 percent of patients, increasing appetite, relieving abdominal distension and improving the results of liver function tests."[58]

Scullcap has widespread use as well for anxiety, depression, insomnia, headaches, cramps, and PMS symptoms.[59] It is shown to have strong anti-arthritic and anti-inflammatory actions, due in part to its high content of flavonoids, compounds which are over 1000 times more potent in action than histamines.[60]

Prepare by bringing water to a boil and steeping 1 teaspoon per cup of water for 5 to 10 minutes. During withdrawal, drink ½ to 1 cup every 2 hours and take with the Ese and Top Formulas for fuller effect.

MINERALS

In December 1945, in the United States Soil Conservation publications, the following statements were made:

"The U.S. produces more food than any other nation in the world, yet, according to Dr. Thomas Parran, Jr., 40 percent of the population suffers from malnutrition. How can this be true? The majority of people get enough to eat. Evidently the food eaten does not have enough of the right minerals and vitamins in it to keep them healthy. What causes food to lack these necessary elements? Investigators have found that food is no richer in minerals than the soil from which it comes. Depleted soils will not produce healthy nutritious plants. Plants suffering from mineral deficiencies will not nourish healthy animals. Mineral-deficient plants and undernourished animals will not support our people in health. Poor soils perpetuate poor people physically, mentally, and financially."[61]

All nutrients such as vitamins, proteins, enzymes, amino acids, carbohydrates, fats, sugars, oils, require minerals for proper cellular function. All bodily processes depend upon the action and presence of minerals. Minerals are more important in nutrition than vitamins. Vitamins are required for every biochemical process in the body, but they cannot function unless minerals are first present.

Minerals are the catalysts that make enzyme functions possible. They combine with enzymes into an alkaline detoxifying agent which neutralizes the acid metabolic by-products of the cells and other toxic conditions within the body and prepares them for elimination. Due to the rapid use and depletion of minerals during tissue rebuilding and detoxification, a saturation of minerals is required for continuation of healing during a health crisis to restore the electrolytic balance needed for effective body electronic functions. Our electrical system cannot work without minerals. A lack of minerals slows down the electronic process and retards healing.

Hormonal secretion of glands is dependent upon mineral stimulation. The acid-alkaline balance (pH) of the tissue fluid is controlled by minerals. Minerals are, therefore, required as supplemental dietary food, especially now when the mineral content of our soil is deficient. Our fruits and vegetables, once mineral-rich, are now void of minerals and are further destroyed by petrochemicals and synthetic fertilizers.

Mezotrace

Mezotrace is an excellent multiple mineral formula that is mined from a deposit of the shells of minute sea creatures. It has a very high level of elemental calcium (325 mg per tablet) and magnesium (200 mg per tablet). It also has good amounts of iron and many trace minerals. All the minerals are in a naturally chelated form so their absorption is excellent. One of the greatest deficiencies people with addictions incur is of calcium and magnesium with resultant nervous system instability, liver deterioration, etc. This formula is excellent for supplying full nourishment of these key elements.

Mezotrace has also been very helpful for people with arthritis, osteoporosis, dental caries, and other illnesses involving mineral depletion. Recommended use is 2 to 4 tablets daily with meals.

Multiple Mineral

A good multiple mineral formula is invaluable to the program of the recovering addict. No multiple mineral formulas contain the high doses of calcium and magnesium that the recovering addict needs, so he or she should take extra calcium and magnesium supplements as well. Among the best quality multiple mineral formulas are the food-grown types made by Grow Co. and distributed by its licensees: Rainbow Light, Lifestar, MegaFood. Schiff has also developed excellent chelated mineral formulations.

Zinc Picolinate

One significant way alcohol, sugar, and caffeine cause liver damage is by leaching out the liver's stores of zinc. Zinc plays an important part in carbohydrate metabolism. Diets high in protein, whole grains, brewer's yeast, eggs, oysters, and pumpkin seeds supply good amounts of zinc. People who do not eat balanced meals and those who use excessive amounts of sugar, caffeine, alcohol, and drugs easily develop zinc deficiencies, which can cause deterioration of the liver, reproductive organs, immune system, and skin. Many cases of eating disorders have cleared up when ample amounts of zinc were added to the diet. Zinc picolinate is the most absorbable form of chelated zinc. Recommended use is 20 mg once or twice daily, or more if severely deficient.

Calcium

Calcium is one of the most important nutrients needed in ample amounts for the recovering addict. Sugar, caffeine, alcohol, and other drugs all cause the body to eliminate calcium. Caffeine has been shown to double the urinary excretion of calcium.[62] Most alcoholics and addicts eat poorly and have an inadequate intake of calcium to begin with. A number of studies have recorded low serum calcium levels in chronic alcoholics.[63]

Low calcium and magnesium levels are a major contributing factor to the irritability, pain, and muscular/nervous system disorders that alcoholics and addicts experience during the withdrawal and recovery phases.

Recovering addicts should take 1000 to 2000 mg elemental calcium in divided doses with meals. Preferably, they should use a good quality chelated mineral formula like Mezotrace, the orotates, or the aspertates.

Magnesium

Magnesium is the other main mineral that, along with calcium, helps maintain a strong and calm nervous system. Sugar, caffeine, alcohol and drugs also contribute to creating a magnesium deficiency. A magnesium deficiency was discovered in chronic alcoholic patients.[64] Low calcium and magnesium levels are a major contributing factor to the irritability, pain, and muscular/ nervous system disorders that alcoholics and addicts experience during withdrawal and recovery phases.

Recovering addicts should use 1000 to 2000 mg a day of magnesium in divided doses with meals. They should preferably use a good quality chelated mineral formula like Mezotrace, the orotates, or the aspertates. Magnesium oxide should not be used, as it can cause severe irritation of the digestive tract.

Iron

Many people today, especially women, suffer from low levels of iron and borderline anemia which may be too marginal to show up on blood tests, and yet may still create a condition of chronic fatigue and weak immune system. The daily amount of iron the average American woman consumes today falls almost a full 40 percent below the RDA, making it the nutrient that is perhaps most lacking in the diet.[65]

Addicts and alcoholics are especially prone to develop anemia because substance abuse can damage the liver and because they frequently have poor eating habits. There are many factors involved in proper assimilation of iron, and a diet high in good quality protein with many additional supportive nutrients may be needed to successfully treat anemia. Among these are Omega 3 fatty acids,[66] copper, vitamin C, and B vitamins.

The best iron supplement by far is Liv.52.[67] Because of the special way the iron is organically complexed and mixed with supportive herbs, its assimilation is very high.

Other good iron supplements are: Food Grown Iron distributed by Lifestar, Rainbow Light, or Mega Food, and the Standard Process Iron formula.

Some iron supplements can be very toxic, especially in the large quantities often prescribed.

Good foods for iron deficiency include: organic liver, oysters, leafy greens, red meat, and beans.

Trace Minerals (Manganese, Molybdenum, and others)

People who have been eating poorly and abusing addictive substances also develop deficiencies of many of the key trace minerals like manganese and molybdenum. Manganese is important in carbohydrate metabolism, nervous system function, and ligament strength. Molybdenum is important in rebuilding the liver and other activities. It is also important in the recovery program to eat amply of foods high in minerals and to use herbs and quality chelated mineral formulas for additional support. Use as directed.

Potassium

Potassium deficiency is one of the most widespread nutritional deficiencies today. Excessive consumption of salt, use of caffeine, alcohol and sugar, and poor dietary habits all contribute to the development of a potassium deficiency. Some pharmaceuticals like Cortisone, Prednisone, and diuretics can also create a potassium deficiency. This deficiency is a major cause of high blood pressure and heart disease, and many scientific studies have established that normalizing potassium intake results in normalizing blood pressure levels.[68] Low potassium levels also weaken adrenal and liver function.

Taking extra potassium daily in the form of fresh fruit and vegetable juices, herbal extracts, or formulations like Km is very helpful for people with potassium deficiencies. Other good sources are potatoes, bananas, leafy green vegetables, oranges, whole grains, and sunflower seeds.

GTF Chromium

GTF (glucose tolerance factor) chromium has an important place in helping to regulate blood sugar levels and metabolize carbohydrates. It also works with growth hormone to build up muscle tissue mass. Consumption of refined sugars and carbohydrates can increase chromium loss up to 300 percent and many diets are already deficient in GTF chromium. There are many types of chromium supplements, but most have very poor assimilation and metabolic capacities. Independent studies at the Linus Pauling Institute Of Science and Medicine ranked Chrome Mate first in the criteria required of a true GTF chromium. Use as directed.

Selenium

Selenium plays a key part in the body's utilization of oxygen. Research studies have found that mice survived longer without oxygen when they were supplemented with selenium.[69] Alcoholics were found to have below normal levels of selenium, and those with liver disease found to have the lowest levels.[70] Heart disease and cancer are higher in people with low selenium levels.[71]

The main function of selenium in humans is as a coenzyme in the enzyme glutathione peroxidase. The function of glutathione peroxidase is to break down hydrogen peroxide. Selenium also has a major part to play in the detoxifying of poisonous phenols, formaldehyde, acetylaldehyde, hydrocarbons, and chlorine. Many people with allergic reactions to these chemicals have received marked improvement through the use of selenium supplementation.

Selenium can be very toxic in excess. People and wildlife have become seriously ill in some parts of the country where the water supply is contaminated with selenium.

The normal safe therapeutic dose is 100 to 200 mcs per day and the best form is from the whole food concentrates.

AMINO ACIDS

DLPA

DL-Phenylalanine is composed of two amino acids, D Phenylalanine and L Phenylalanine. This formula works to extend the lifespan of endorphins by slowing down their destruction by certain endorphin-chewing enzymes. It also is the raw material the nervous system uses to make PEA (Phenylethylamine) which increases the body's capacity to utilize endorphins, and triggers the release of some endorphins.[72]

Use of DLPA is especially indicated for recovering cocaine and stimulant addicts, because it helps to rebuild the norepinephrine levels which are depleted by the drug use.

DLPA is especially useful in reducing cravings in the recovering addict and also in helping clear up the depression, pain, and nervous system instability experienced as the body rebuilds. One double-blind study by Dr. Heller compared the effect of D Phenylalanine with imipramine, the most commonly prescribed tricyclic antidepressant, for 60 patients. Those given D Phenyla-lanine had a higher rate of improvement, without the side effects of the antidepressant.[73]

DLPA has also been used successfully in nutritional programs for arthritis.

Recommended dose is 750 mg to 1000 mg twice daily with meals.

Glutamine

Glutamine, a "non-essential" amino acid, improves intelligence and helps control hypoglycemia and the craving for alcohol and sweets. It also helps fatigue and improves the healing of ulcers. The brain uses only two substances for fuel, sugar and glutamine, so increasing the amount of glutamine in the diet improves nervous system function.

Dr. Roger Williams has done extensive research with glutamine and found that regular use greatly reduced cravings for alcohol and sweets in alcoholics and sugar addicts. Dr. Abram Hoffer has used glutamine with other nutrients in successful programs for people with schizophrenia, senility, and mental retardation. Other researchers like Janice Keller, M.D., have found it effective against drug addiction as well as alcohol and sugar cravings. Recommended use is 1000 mg, 2 or 3 times daily, or more for severe conditions.

VITAMINS

Vitamin C

Many authorities find vitamin C to be among the most essential ingredients in the treatment of addiction. Vitamin C is a primary detoxifier of drugs and poisons from the system. It also helps neutralize much of the withdrawal difficulties, and it is powerful in rebuilding the liver, adrenals, and immune system.

Libby and Stone (1977) and Libby, et al, (1982, a,b,c) reported that large doses of ascorbic acid combined with B vitamins and protein allowed heroin addicts to quit without withdrawal symptoms. They were then given daily maintenance doses (10 grams) which prevented all cravings for heroin. Free and Sanders (1978) corroborated their results.

Ascorbic acid, the synthetic form of vitamin C, is highly acidic, and when used in moderate or large doses can cause ulceration of the digestive tract and further depletion of calcium and magnesium levels in many people. It is best to use the form that is buffered with calcium and magnesium, the ester C, or the food-complexed vitamin C developed by Grow Company.

Vitamin B Complex

The importance of the B complex vitamins in the recovery process is enormous, and volumes of books, as well as large numbers of research studies, have been done on them. This is just a brief review of the most important information, and the reader is encouraged to seek out more extensive literature on the subject.

It is a well-known fact that people who use excessive amounts of sugar, caffeine, alcohol and drugs develop serious B vitamin deficiencies which adverseley affect their mental and physical well being. What is not so well known is that many of these people had B vitamin deficiencies before they became addicted, and that these deficiencies can create cravings for addictive substances. The *British Journal of Addiction* cited experiments in Finland where rats made deficient in B vitamins were more likely to choose alcohol than water when both were placed before them. Supplementing their diets with B vitamins reversed their taste, and they began choosing water over alcohol.

Bill Wilson, Co-Founder of Alcoholics Anonymous, Dr. Russel Smith, Dr. Abram Hoffer, Dr. Janice Phelps, Dr. Roger Williams, Dr. Carl Pfeiffer and many other physicians have found B vitamins of immeasurable value in the recovery process of many addicts. Use of B vitamins has been found to greatly diminish or eliminate withdrawal symptoms, help clear up cravings, significantly improve mental outlook and stability, and aid regeneration of the liver, endocrine glands, and nervous system.

Bill Wilson first tried using niacin supplements on himself and, observing their beneficial effects, gave them to 30 of his associates in AA who also were helped.[74] Medical researchers have found that niacin (vitamin B3) and pantothenic acid (vitamin B5) greatly facilitate the breakdown and elimination of acetylaldehyde, so that it does not end up as THIQ. THIQ, a chemical produced in the brains of alcoholics, is more than 500 times stronger than morphine, and causes people to crave and become addicted to alcohol. Dr. Russel Smith completed studies on thousands of patients using niacin with excellent results.[75] Because of severe liver damage and other factors, many people do not tolerate synthetic niacin, niacinimide, or other B vitamin supplements, and need to work with diet, liver supplements, brewer's yeast, and herbal formulas to restore their health.

Vitamin E

Vitamin E is a powerful antioxidant and helps the body break down poisons. It also greatly increases oxygen supplies to the cells. Vitamin E nourishes and increases the production of adrenal and reproductive hormones and strengthens the immune system. It also improves nervous system function, and has been shown to help restore the function of damaged livers.[76] Vitamin E helps varicose veins, the circulatory system, and the heart. The natural, not synthetic, form of alpha tocopherol has been shown to have the most nutritional and biological value. Recommended use is 400 to 1000 I.U. natural D-Alpha Tocopherol daily with meals.

Vitamin A

Vitamin A is an important vitamin for recovering addicts for several reasons. Many alcoholics and addicts have developed a deficiency of vitamin A, which aids regeneration of the liver and other tissues. Poor liver and thyroid functions make many addicts unable to convert the beta carotene form into vitamin A.

The best form to take is either fish oil concentrate capsules which contain 10,000 to 25,000 I.U. vitamin A and 1000 I.U. vitamin D or Emulsified Cod Liver Oil which will also supply needed Omega 3 fatty acids.

BENEFICIAL DIGESTIVE FLORAS

A complete colonization of the digestive tract with all the beneficial intestinal floras is an essential part of a healthy functioning human body. A normal adult has three types of beneficial intestinal floras: streptococcus faecium, acidophilus, and bifidus. These bacteria are essential for human life. They help digest food, produce vitamins, and are a key factor in the body's control of pathogenic yeast, bacteria, viruses, and parasites. They also provide other important but as yet unknown functions in the immune system.

Each of the three floras has distinct and critical functions, and an imbalance or deficiency in one can severely affect the functioning of the organism as a whole. For example, bifidus breaks down lactose, or milk sugar; a deficiency causes an inability to digest dairy products. In healthy infants, bifidus colonies make up 80 percent of their beneficial flora.[77]

Abundant colonization of the digestive tract with these three floras is one of the main homeostatic mechanisms the body has for controlling the growth and infection of pathogenic organisms. Proper colonization can be damaged by many things. The most common are stress, negative emotions, poor diet (lack of fiber and use of excessively refined and simple carbohydrates), and use of antibiotics, antiparasite medications, steroids, and birth control pills.

Proper implantation of all three floras is a foundation block of any holistic yeast recovery program. The quickest and most effective method is to ingest large amounts orally.

There are several companies making good quality acidophilus, bifidus, and streptococcus faecium formulas.

Those who suffer severe yeast infection of the digestive tract need to take the floras continuously in order to gain control. This can take a few weeks or up to a couple of years, depending on the individual and the severity of infection.

An important part of any vaginal infection treatment is vaginal implantation of acidophilus. Douche with a 20 percent solution of apple cider vinegar. Mix one-half to 1 teaspoon of acidophilus in a small amount of warm water, then implant.

Regular consumption of good quality sauerkraut, pickles and yogurt is another important part of the flora replenishing program.

For those without dairy allergies, the best method of implanting large colonies of flora is to culture your own yogurt from one of the three floras and eat half a cup with a one or two meals daily.

Some of the best brands of Flora are: Jarrow Formulas, Meta-Genics or Ethical Nutrients, SISU, Sunrider, and Yerba Prima.

ENZYMES

S.O.D.

The fact that this is the fifth most abundant enzyme the body produces says a lot. S.O.D. has a major part to play in oxidation in the metabolic cycles within the liver to break down poisons. Recovering addicts will find this very helpful in aiding liver detoxification of poisons, thereby greatly relieving withdrawal symptoms. It also has been found to help break down toxins in joints that can cause arthritic symptoms. Only in the past few years has research into its properties been done, and I feel the future will bring a great deal more evidence to show its critical place in many metabolic processes.

S.O.D. is one of the foremost enzymes the body uses to break down free radicals. This is especially important today, as the tremendous increase in poisons from drugs, environmental toxins, and toxins in foods create much greater amounts of free radicals in our tissues, which in turn are implicated as major causative factors in degenerative diseases like arthritis and cancer.

The best S.O.D. is made by Biomed foods in Hawaii. They are the only company that makes S.O.D. tablets in the millions of units. Take 4 to 6 tablets daily for the first month or two, then decrease to 2 or 3 a day.

WITHDRAWAL

The withdrawal phase is the most difficult and painful part of recovery. The symptoms can be as simple as headaches, irritability, and fatigue for the mildly addicted, to delirium tremens with hallucinations, which may require sedation and physical restraint, for the hard core addict.

Doctors have found that use of large amounts of vitamin C (up to 1 gram per hour), calcium and magnesium (1 gram every 6 hours), plenty of fluids, glutamine, B vitamins, and frequent meals with high protein foods combined with flax seed oil greatly ease the difficulties of this phase.

Many people have also found that frequent drinks of herbal teas taken with NuPlus, Flax Seed Oil, GLA, Ginseng, Prime Again, Action Caps, Quinary, Top, Ese, Liv.52, Miso, and nutritional yeast greatly facilitated breaking out of the addiction cycle.

It is not possible in these pages to provide a separate protocol for the myriad addictive conditions: from the simple dependence on a little sugar or coffee to the severe addiction to alcohol, hard drugs, or barbiturates. One good approach is to begin using a large amount of the formulas listed in the "Protocol For Continued Nutritional Support" and eating well for several weeks, to build up nutritional reserves and basic strength while trying to quit. Many people have found that once they began using these formulas and eating well, their addictive cravings went away and it was easy for them to quit.

Working with AA or a similar 12-step program has also proven helpful to many people. It is strongly recommended that those with serious addictions find a holistic doctor or medical center and support groups to work with them when attempting to quit. There is a list of facilities in the back of this book.

SAMPLE PROTOCOL

For Continued Nutritional Support
For First Several Months Of Recovery
Or Building Up Health In Exhausted Co-Dependent

First Thing In The Morning
Herb tea or glass of water
¼ to ½ teaspoon or 2 to 3 capsules Glutamine
2 capsules each Top and Ese

20 Minutes Later
Herb tea with 30 drops Milk Thistle Extract or 2 tablets Milk
     Thistle
6 Prime Again capsules
(Alpha 20C, Lifestream, Ginseng, and Action Caps, if
     needed)

With Breakfast
2 Mezotrace or similar high potency calcium-magnesium
     formula
1 teaspoon Flax Seed Oil
1 Beauty Pearl
1 Zinc Picolinate
1 to 2 Quinary packets
100 to 500 mg Vitamin C
400 to 1000 IU Vitamin E
1 to 4 tablets multiple vitamin mineral
2 to 3 tablets Liv.52
1 Super GLA capsule or 3 to 4 capsules Omega Plus

3 Hours After Breakfast
Herbal tea or water

Half Hour Later
Tea or water with 1 to 3 teaspoons NuPlus and 30 drops
Milk Thistle Extract or 3 tablets Milk Thistle

With Lunch
1 Vitamin B Complex if needed

3 Hours After Lunch
Herbal tea

Half Hour Later
Tea with 1 to 3 teaspoons NuPlus and 30 drops Milk
Thistle Extract or 3 tables Milk Thistle
6 Prime Again
¼ to ½ teaspoon or 2 to 3 capsules Glutamine
(Action Caps, Lifestream, and Alpha 20C, if needed)

With Dinner
2 Mezotrace or similar high potency calcium-magnesium
formula
1 teaspoon Flax Seed Oil
2 capsules DL Phenylalanine
1 Zinc Picolinate
100 to 500 mg Vitamin C
1 to 2 Quinary packets
2 to 3 Liv.52 tablets
1 Super GLA capsule or 3 capsules Omega Plus

Bedtime
Chamomile Tea
2 capsules each Ese and Top

Herbal Teas can be taken throughout the day, as desired.

Also, supplemental "super foods" such as Bee Pollen, Algae, Green Magma, and Brewer's Yeast may be taken with meals for additional support.

Note: After 1 to 3 months, the GLA or Omega Plus can sometimes be eliminated and the Flax Seed Oil continued at a maintenance dosage of 1 to 3 teaspoons daily.

BASIC NUTRITIONAL PROTOCOL

First Thing In Morning
Glass warm water sipped slowly
Herbal tea

With Breakfast:
Calcium Magnesium formula (Mezotrace, etc.)
Multimineral
Vitamin C
1 to 3 teaspoons Flax Seed Oil
Vitamin E (Natural Alpha Tocopherol)
2 Liv.52 tablets
Strengthening herbs as desired

Half Hour Before Lunch
Herbal tea

Half Hour Before Dinner
Herbal tea

With Dinner
Calcium Magnesium formula (Mezotrace, etc.)
Multimineral
Zinc Picolinate
Vitamin C
2 Liv.52 tablets
Strengthening herbs

Bedtime
Herbal tea

Optional supplementation with Herbal Formulas, B Complex, Nutritional Yeast and/or NuPlus may be taken with meals for additional support.

SAMPLE PROTOCOL

For Those Who Want
A Very Simple Program or
Those With a Limited Budget

First Thing In The Morning
Herb Tea

With Breakfast:
Vitamin C
1 to 3 teaspoons Flax Seed Oil
2 Mezotrace (or 500 mg elemental calcium and 500 mg
    elemental magnesium in
chelated form)
2 Liv.52 tablets

Half Hour Later
Tea (same as above)

Mid Morning
NuPlus

Half Hour Before Lunch
Tea (same as above)

Half Hour After Lunch
Tea (same as above)

Mid Afternoon
NuPlus

Half Hour Before Dinner
Tea (same as above)

With Dinner
Vitamin C
1 Zinc Picolinate
2 Mezotrace (or 500 mg elemental calcium and 500 m
    elemental magnesium in chelated form)
2 Liv.52 tablets

Half Hour After Dinner
Tea (same as above)

Before Bed
Herbal Relaxing Tea: Chamomile, Scullcap, etc.

The main features of this program are to eat regular, good meals with lots of protein and vegetables. Eat lots of eggs, fish, and nutritional yeast, if tolerated. Avoid sugar, refined and processed foods, etc.

Make up 1 to 2 quarts of tea and drink throughout the day. (A thermos can be taken to work if necessary.)

Chamomile tea can be taken, if needed, to calm the nerves or soothe the stomach.

SAMPLE PROTOCOL

For Those With
High Histamine Levels (Histadelia)

First Thing In The Morning:
Glass of warm water—sipped slowly
Cup Herb Tea
6 S.O.D. tablets—Biomed Foods

With Breakfast
   2 Mezotrace
   1 Beauty Pearl
   30 to 50 mg Coenzyme Q10
   Vitamin C
   1 Super GLA Capsule or 3 Omega Plus capsules
   500 to 1000 I.U. Natural Alpha Tocopherol Vitamin E
   1 teaspoon Flax Seed Oil
   3 Conco
   2 Prime Again
   2 Alpha 20C
   3 Milk Thistle Extract & Concentrate
   2 to 3 Liv.52 tablets

Mid Morning
   Herbal tea
   1 to 3 teaspoons NuPlus

Half Hour Before Lunch
   Herbal tea

With Lunch
   1 Mezotrace
   1 Zinc Picolinate
   50 mg Pyridoxal Phosphate Coenzyme Vitamin B6
   1 Coenzyme Q10
   1 Chelated Manganese
   Vitamin C

Mid Afternoon
   Herbal tea

Half Hour Before Dinner:
   Herbal tea

With Dinner
1 Mezotrace
1 Zinc Picolinate
1 Chelated Manganese
1 Super GLA Capsule or 3 Omega Plus capsules
1 teaspoon Flax Seed Oil
200 mg Chelated Calcium
3 Conco
2 Prime Again
2 Alpha 20C
3 Milk Thistle Extract & Concentrate
2 to 3 Liv.52

Bedtime
Tea: Chamomile, Valerian Root, Marigold, Catnip (any one or combination)

Additional formulas that have been found to help reduce high histamine levels are: Quercitin (1000 to 2000 mg daily), Prime Again (4 to 8 more capsules daily), Conco (4 to 6 more capsules daily), Alpha 20 C (4 to 8 capsules daily), NuPlus (1 to 3 teaspoon used 1 to 3 times daily), Calli tea, B vitamins, thyroid support, adrenal support, chamomile tea and scullcap tea.

It is often important to identify those foods to which one is allergic and eliminate them from the diet, as well identify the sources of any environmental allergens and eliminate them as much as is practical.

After 1 to 3 months, the GLA or Omega Plus capsules can sometimes be eliminated and the Flax Seed Oil kept at a maintenance dosage of 1 to 3 teaspoons daily.

This is a very full program for people with severely high histamine and/or allergic conditions. As the condition improves, usually within a few months, the program can be simplified. Also, for mild or moderate conditions the amounts of formulas and dosages can be reduced significantly.

As always, these are general guidelines. Each individual is unique and needs to discover the appropriate amounts of formulas suited to his/her condition.

HEALING BULIMIA AND COMPULSIVE EATING

Identify any underlying disorders such as zinc deficiency, iron deficiency, Omega 3 fatty acid deficiency, underactive thyroid, adrenal or ovarian function, or yeast overgrowth.

Formulas that have been found to help this condition are: Liv.52, NuPlus, Calli Tea, Beauty Pearl, Action Caps, Prime Again, Flax Seed Oil, B vitamins, zinc picolinate, and digestive floras. The yeast disorder program is also very helpful, for those who have yeast overgrowth, and endocrine glandular support is indicated for people with these disorders.

HEALING THE FOOD ALLERGY ADDICTION SYNDROME

Identify existing food allergies using the food specific IgC Antibody Test or fasting and food elimination approach. Identify any existing nutritional deficiencies, endocrine glandular weakness, or yeast overgrowth syndrome. Establish a good diet or nutritional program.

Formulas that have been found to help this condition are: vitamin C, B vitamins, zinc picolinate, Liv.52, Calli tea, Fortune Delight tea, Prime Again, Beauty Pearl, Action Caps, NuPlus, Flax Seed Oil, GLA, and Alpha 20C. The yeast disorder program is also very helpful, as well as endocrine glandular support.

The most revealing, up-to-date, and extensive presentation on the causes of and therapies for food allergy, addiction, and essential fatty acid and prostaglandin deficiencies is found in the recent book *Essential Fatty Acids and Immunity In Mental Health*, by Charles Bates, published by Life Science Press.

Endnotes to Chapter 8

1. Phelps, Janice Keller, M.D. and Alan E. Nourse, M.D.,*The Hidden Addiction and How To Get Free* (Boston: Little, Brown & Co., 1986).

2. Shurtleff, William, *The Book of Miso* (Berkeley, CA: Ten Speed Press, 1982).

3. Hamaker, John D., *The Survival of Civilization* (California: Hamaker-Weaver, 1982).

4. Gittleman, Ann Louise, M.S., *Beyond Pritikin* (New York: Bantam, 1988).

5. Ballentine, Rudolph, M.D., "Butter vs. Oil," IN *East/West Journal* (February 1988).

6. Rudin, Donald O., M.D. and Clara Felix, *The Omega 3 Phenomenon* (New York: Rawson Associates, 1987); Bates, Charles, Ph.D., *Essential Fatty Acids and Immunity in Mental Health* (Washington: Life Science Press, 1987); and Finnegan, John, *Understanding Oils and Fats* (California: Elysian Arts, 1990).

7. Galli, Claudio and Artemis P. Simopoulos, *Dietary Omega 3 and Omega 6 Fatty Acids: Biological Effects and Nutritional Essentiality* (New York and London: Plenum Press, 1989).

8. Swern, Daniel, Ed., *Bailey's Industrial Oil and Fat Products* (New York: John Wiley and Sons, 1979).

9. Gittleman, op cit.

10. Finnegan, op cit.

11. Gittlemen, op cit.

12. Finnegan, op cit.

13. Ibid.

14. Gittleman, op cit.

15. Finnegan, op cit.

16. Ibid.

17. Rudin, op cit.

18. Bates, op cit.

19. Finnegan, op cit.

20. Rudin, op cit.

21. Finnegan, op cit.

22. Bates, op cit.

23. Finnegan, op cit.

24. Atoba, M.A., E.A. Ayoola, and O. Ogunseyinde, "Effect of Essential Phospholipid Choline on the Course of Acute Hepatitis-B In-

fection," IN *Topical Gastroenterology* 6(2) (April-June 1985), pages 96-99.

25. Jenkins, P.J., B. P. Portmann, A.L.W.F. Eddleston, and R. Williams, "Use of Polyunsaturated Phosphatidyl Choline in HBsAg Negative Chronic Active Hepatitis: Results of Prospective Double-Blind Controlled Trial,[c1 *Liver 2* (1982) pages 77-81.

26. Kosina, F., K. Budka, Z. Kolouch, D. Lazarova, and D. Truksova, "Essential Cholinephospholipids in the Treatment of Virus Hepatitis" *Casopis Lekaru Ceskych* 120 (31-32) (August 13, 1981), pages 957-960.

27. Visco, G., "Polyunsaturated Phosphatidylcholine in Association with Vitamin B Complex in the Treatment of Acute Viral Hepatitis B: Results of a Randomized Double-Blind Study" *Clinica Terapeutica 114* (3) (August 15, 1985) pages 183-188.

28. Asai, Kazuhiko, *Miracle Cure: Organic Germanium* (Japan Publications, USA, 1980).

29. Bliznakov, Emile G., M.D. and Gerald L. Hunt, *The Miracle Nutrient Coenzyme Q10* (New York: Bantam, 1987).

30. *Liv. 52: A Monograph,* a compilation of over 100 laboratory studies published by the Himalaya Drug Co., Bombay, India.

31. Ibid.

32. Ibid.

33. Ibid.

34. Ibid.

35. Ibid.

36. Ibid.

37. Wren, R.C., F.L.S., *Potter's New Cyclopaedia of Botanical Drugs and Preparations* (C.W. Daniel Co., Ltd., 1988).

38. Murray, Pizzorno J., *A Textbook of Natural Medicine* (Seattle, WA: John Bastyr College Publications, 1987).

39. Murray, Michael, N.D., *Phyto-Pharmica Review* (Fall 1987).

40. Lapis, K., A. Jeney, A. Divald, *et al.*, "Experimental Studies on the Effect of Hepatoprotective Compounds," IN *Tokai Journal of Experimental Clinical Medicine* 11 (Suppl): 135-45 (1986).

41. Graham, Judy, *Evening Primrose Oil* (New York: Thorsons, 1984).

42. Bates, op cit.

43. Ibid.

44. Ibid.

45. Rudin, op cit.

46. Wren, op cit.

47. People who are extremely sensitive to caffeine may have trouble with these teas and can use other herbal teas like Calendula or Milk Thistle Seed instead.

48. Studies performed by the following: University of Scranton; University of Missouri; New Jersey College of Medicine and Dentistry; Reims University, France; and the Brain Bio-Center in New Jersey.

49. Murray, Dr. Michael, N.D., *The 21st Century Herbal* (Washington: Vita-Line, Inc.)

50. Treben, Maria, *Health Through God's Pharmacy* (Austria: Wilhelm Ennsthaler, Steyr, 1987).

51. Moore, Richard D., M.D., Ph.D. and George Webb, Ph.D., *The K Factor* (New York: Pocket Books, 1986).

52. Murray, Michael T., N.D., *Phyto Pharmica Review*, Vol. 1, No. 2 (February 1988).

53. From *Food and Cosmetics Toxicology*, Volume 15 (1977).

54. Murray, op cit.

55. Tierra, Michael, C.A., N.D., *Planetary Herbology* (New Mexico: Lotus Press, 1988).

56. Mabey, Richard, *The New Age Herbalist* (New York: Collier Books, 1988).

57. Ibid.

58. Wren, op cit.

59. Mabey, op cit.; Wren, op cit; Tierra, op cit.; Murray, op cit.

60. Murray, op cit.; Wren, op cit.

61. Manahan, William, M.D., *Eat for Health* (California: H.J. Kramer, 1988).

62. Werbach, Melvyn R., M.D., *Nutritional Influences on Illness* (California: Third Line Press, 1987).

63. Ibid.

64. Phelps, op cit.

65. Stockman, J.A., *Journal of the American Medical Association* 258: 1645-1647 (September 1987)

66. *Liv.52: A Monograph*, op cit.

67. Moore, Richard, op cit.

68. Ibid.

69. Ibid.

70. Werbach, op cit.

71. Werbach, op cit.; Kirschmann, John D. and Lavon J. Dunne, *Nutrition Almanac* (New York: McGraw-Hill, 1984).

72. Ibid.

73. Hoffer, Abram, M.D., Ph.D., *Orthomolecular Medicine for Physicians* (Connecticut: Keats, 1989).

74. Ibid.

75. Ibid.

76. Kirschmann, op cit.

77. A personal anecdote illustrates the uniquely essential function of the individual flora. The six-month-old son of a friend suffered from chronic problems from birth with digesting his mother's milk, with stomach pains, diarrhea, recurrent ear infections, and sore throats. We started him on bifidus flora and all symptoms disappeared within the first day. He no longer spat up the milk, the diarrhea stopped, and he became a much happier baby.

CHAPTER 9
Diet

Proper diet and nutrition are essential elements in a recovery program. Foods are the building blocks the body uses to build healthy organs and the nervous system, and to keep them strong and functioning properly.

The human body is made of five basic classes of nutrients: protein, carbohydrates, fats, vitamins, and minerals. A regular intake of adequate amounts of all nutrients is essential for proper physical and mental health. Most substance abusers have developed serious nutritional deficiencies of key proteins, fats, vitamins, and minerals, and they usually have a disturbed carbohydrate metabolism. This is a major cause of their addictive cravings, withdrawal symptoms, fatigue, depression, irritability, mental derangement, and other conditions.

Practitioners working with recovering addicts have repeatedly found that these people become well—much quicker with far fewer symptoms—and stay drug free much longer when they follow principles of good nutrition. Most substance abusers need three square meals a day with good quality protein, complex carbohydrates, and fats served at each meal. They often need snacks as well, especially during the early stages of recovery.

Rebuilding damaged livers, tissues, nervous systems, and glands requires more protein, vitamins, minerals, and Omega 3 fatty acids than those required by healthy people. Also, since they invariably have an inability to handle simple carbohydrates properly, addicts need to avoid the simple sugars, and use fruits and fruit juices only moderately. Ample amounts of complex carbohydrates, such as beans, grains, and potatoes are needed. Good sources of protein are fish, chicken, meat, eggs, beans, cheese, nuts, and seeds.

Good quality fats are also essential elements in a well-balanced diet. Just as our bodies need protein, carbohydrates, calcium, and other nutrients for good health and proper functioning, we also need certain of the fatty acids. While an excess of fats, especially poor quality fats like hydrogenated oils, contributes to disease, an inadequate dietary intake of fats also can cause ill health.

There are two main classes of fats—saturated and unsaturated. Our bodies need a minimum amount (20 to 30 percent of calories) of both types of fats. The best sources of saturated fats are butter, dairy products, eggs, fowl, and meats. While excessive amounts of cholesterol are harmful, we need a minimal amount, as it is a main nutrient used in the building of our nerves, skin, steroid hormones, and other major body components.

The unsaturated fats are mostly made up of the Omega 3 and Omega 6 fatty acids. These also are essential to the normal health of the human organism. While many people in industrialized nations tend to get adequate amounts of the Omega 6 (linoleic acid) fatty acid, and some get excessive amounts which can contribute to disease, most are seriously deficient in the vital Omega 3 (alpha-linolenic acid) fatty acid.[1, 2, 3, 4]

Our bodies use the Omega 3 and Omega 6 fatty acids to produce energy and heat, and to produce the essential prostaglandins, hormone-like substances which help regulate the immune system, glandular, and nervous system functioning. The Omega 6 fatty acids are the raw materials the body uses to produce gamma linolenic acid (GLA) which has been shown to have great value in treating the recovering addict-alcoholic. These are just a few of the key functions these fats play in nourishing health and preventing disease.

Flax seed oil is the highest source of the Omega 3 fatty acids, and a good source of the Omega 6 fatty acid. It is good tasting and can be poured directly onto protein dishes, vegetables, salads, grains, soups, etc. Adults need 1 to 3 teaspoons of flax seed oil daily or to eat fatty fish several times a week to receive an adequate amount of the Omega 3 fatty acid.[3] The best sources of properly produced and packaged unrefined oils are Omega Nutrition, Arrowhead Mills/OmegaFlo, Flora Inc., and Galaxy Enterprises.

It's easy to skip meals or grab some fast food or a candy bar, but getting exhausted or going hungry puts stress on the body and nervous system. Fad or starvation diets also will wreak havoc on anyone who is serious about his or her health. Wholesome snacking during the day keeps blood sugar levels stable, and it's easy to keep some nutritional "treats" handy.

Plan balanced meals that include a source of protein, some complex carbohydrates, lots of fresh vegetables and good quality fats.

What foods you select and how they are prepared are very important. Always use fresh vegetables, fruits, whole grains, fish, poultry, and meats. If you can find them, use organic produce and meats, as these are free of harmful antibiotics and pesticides. Avoid processed, frozen or canned foods, as these are missing some of the key nutritional elements.

When you eat out, eat selectively, avoiding fried and junk foods. Most chicken and meats (with the exception of lamb) contain antibiotics and hormones. However, many restaurants have a fresh catch of the day, which you can order baked or broiled, along with a potato or rice, salad, and vegetables. A potato or rice with vegetables and salad can also be sufficient on occasion. You can afford to skip the dessert. Most commercial desserts are made from refined sugar and flour, which for some people are very hard to digest, cause too rapid a change in blood sugar levels, and put a lot of stress on the pancreas and liver.

The best methods for cooking are lightly sauteing, steaming, baking, and broiling. When sauteing, use a small amount of raw butter, extra virgin olive oil, or unrefined hazelnut, safflower, sunflower, or sesame oil. It is recommended that one use quality brands mentioned previously. These can be found in most health food stores. Margarine and processed fats have been shown to be severely harmful to health. Use a low to medium heat, so that the oil does not get too hot, making it rancid and very difficult for the body to digest. If you add a small amount of water when sauteing, you will find that vegetables cook more quickly, while keeping the temperature down so the fat does not burn.

To steam vegetables, put them in a pot with about an inch of purified water in the bottom. Bring it to a boil, then lower the heat, so the vegetables gently simmer. When the vegetables are done, do not throw the water away, as it contains lots of nutrients from the vegetables. It can be used as a stock for soup or drunk as a broth. This broth is best if it was made from a purified or distilled water. Most tap waters contain toxins and chemicals that are damaging to one's health. There is a wide range of good quality water filters available. If you use distilled water, it is a good idea to replenish trace minerals by eating seaweed or by taking a good mineral supplement.

Cooking can be fun and a great creative outlet, and it is easy to prepare delicious, well-balanced meals quickly. You can make a pot of rice, for example, which can be eaten throughout the week, either plain, sauteed with vegetables, or added to soups to make them a meal in themselves. Once you get used to preparing and eating only good quality fresh foods, it will be difficult to settle for less.

Preparing food for yourself is one of the ways in which you can truly love and honor yourself as a human being. Often addicts and co-dependents suffer from feelings of guilt and un-worthiness. By learning how to take care of your body, you can help build precious self-esteem that can permeate other aspects of your life. Every meal can be another step towards a balanced, healthy life.

Eat slowly, and chew your food well, so that your body will get maximum benefit from the food. Life is precious, and this is your chance to make a new start every day, to recover from your illness and regain your strength, vitality, and happiness.

For more information, see *Natural Foods and Good Cooking*, by John Finnegan and Kathy Cituk.

Endnotes to Chapter 9

1. Cituk, Kathy and John Finnegan, *Natural Foods and Good Cooking* (California: Elysian Arts, 1989).

2. Rudin, Donald O., M.D. and Clara Felix, *The Omega 3 Phenomenon* (New York: Rawson Associates, 1987).

3. Gittleman, Ann Louise, M.S., *Beyond Pritikin* (New York: Bantam, 1988).

4. Finnegan, John, *Understanding Oils and Fats* (California: Elysian Arts, 1990).

CHAPTER 10

Recipes

Here are a few simple recipes:

Chicken Vegetable Soup

1 boneless breast of chicken
   cut into pieces
1 tbs. butter
4 cups water
1 cup chopped onion
1 tsp. minced garlic
3 thin slices fresh ginger
½ cup sliced carrots
½ cup sliced celery
½ cup green beans

1 cup pea pods
½ cup diced green bell pepper
½ cup diced red bell pepper
½ cup cabbage
1 bay leaf
2 tsp. ground cumin
2 tsp. ground coriander
1 tsp. curry powder (optional)
salt and pepper to taste

Put butter, chicken, onion, garlic, ginger, and spices in soup pot with water. Bring to boil and simmer for 15 minutes. Add carrots, green beans, and green bell pepper. Continue to simmer for 5 minutes. Add red bell pepper, pea pods, and cabbage, and simmer for an additional 3 minutes or until vegetables are tender. Serves 2.

Fish and/or Shrimp Stew

your favorite fish, cut into
   pieces
fresh peeled shrimp
1 tbs. butter
1 cup water
1 cup chopped onion
1 tsp. minced garlic
3 slices fresh ginger
2 tsp. ground cumin
2 tsp. ground coriander or
   ¼ cup fresh chopped
   coriander

¼ tsp. each ground
   fenugreek, nutmeg, and
   cinnamon (optional)
salt and pepper to taste
1 cup chopped potatoes
1 cup pea pods
1 cup green beans
½ cup sliced carrots
2 cups chopped greens (kale,
   chard or cabbage)
½ cup diced red bell pepper

Put fish, shrimp, butter, water, onion, garlic, ginger, and spices in large skillet. Saute about 15 minutes, add potatoes, peas, green beans, and carrots, and continue to saute for another 5 minutes. Add more water if necessary. Add greens and red bell pepper and saute for another 3 minutes. Serves 2.

Lamb Stew

Lamb is one of the nicest meats to use. All lamb is range fed and is free of antibiotics and added hormones.

2 lamb chops, fat trimmed
   and cut into pieces
1 tbs. butter
1 cup chopped onion
1 tsp. minced garlic
3 slices fresh ginger
1 tsp. ground cumin
1 tsp. ground coriander
¼ tsp. cumin seeds
¼ tsp. celery seeds
1 tsp. curry powder
pinch cayenne

salt and pepper to taste
½ cup corn sliced from cob
   (optional)
1 cup diced potatoes
1 cup sliced carrots
1 cup sliced celery
1 cup broccoli
½ cup diced red bell pepper
½ cup chopped cabbage
2 quartered tomatoes
   (optional)

Put lamb, oil, onion, garlic, ginger, corn, and spices in a skillet with small amount of water. Simmer about 15 minutes, and add potatoes, carrots, celery, and tomatoes and continue to simmer for about 5 minutes. Add remaining vegetables and simmer for another 3 minutes. Serves two.

Easy Vegetable Soup

2 cups water
½ cup chopped onion
½ tsp. minced garlic
3 slices fresh ginger

½ cup sliced carrots
½ cup sliced celery
½ cup chopped cabbage
½ cup sliced zucchini

Put water, onion, garlic, carrots, and celery in pot with salt & pepper. Bring to boil and simmer for 3 minutes. Add cabbage and zucchini and continue to simmer for 3 minutes.

Tasty Lentil Soup

1 cup lentils
3 cups water
1 tbs. butter
½ cup diced onion
1 tsp. chopped garlic
1 bay leaf
¼ tsp. basil
¼ tsp. oregano
¼ tsp. cumin seeds
3 slices fresh ginger

½ cup chopped fresh parsley
  (optional)
½ cup sliced celery
1 cup diced carrots
½ cup chopped green pepper
1 cup chopped tomatoes
  (optional)
salt (or soy sauce) and pepper
  to taste

Rinse lentils thoroughly, then soak in water overnight. Heat lentils, butter, onions, garlic, ginger, parsley, and spices until they boil, then lower heat and simmer for about 1 hour or until lentils are tender. Add the vegetables and tomatoes, and continue to simmer about 10 minutes.

Liver & Onions

Organic liver is one of the best foods to eat when liver function is damaged or weakened.

¼ lb. organic liver
1 cup chopped onion
3 slices fresh ginger
1 tsp. minced garlic

1 cup sliced mushrooms
(optional)
1 tbs. butter

Saute all ingredients together over a medium heat for about 7 minutes. Serves one.

Rice, Millet, Quinoa or Buckwheat

1 cup brown rice, millet, quinoa or buckwheat

2 cups water
½ tsp. salt (optional)

Combine ingredients in pot. Bring to boil, and allow to simmer until water disappears and grain is tender. (Note: Soaking grains overnight in water improves their flavor and makes them easier to digest.)

Try combining grains to enhance their flavor. Half wild rice and half brown rice is my favorite combination. Also, spices such as curry powder, cumin, coriander, and garlic can be added to water and cooked into the grains to make them more flavorful and easier to digest.

Sauteed Rice & Vegetables

1 cup cooked rice (or other grain)
1 tbs. butter
1 cup onion chopped
1 tsp. minced garlic
3 slices fresh ginger
1 tsp. curry powder
(optional)

½ cup sliced carrots
½ cup pea pods
½ cup cabbage
½ cup diced red bell pepper
½ cup sliced zucchini
1 cup chard or kale
Salt and pepper or soy sauce
to taste

Put butter, onion, garlic, ginger, carrots, and spices in skillet with small amount of water and saute for 5 minutes. Add rice and other vegetables and continue to saute for another 3-5 minutes. Serves 2.

Potato & Vegetable Curry

1 tbs. butter
1 cup chopped onion
1 tsp. minced garlic
3 slices fresh ginger
1 cup diced potatoes
   (with skins)
1 cup green beans
½ cup sliced carrots
½ cup pea pods

½ cup diced red bell pepper
½ cup chopped cabbage
½ cup sliced zucchini or
   yellow squash
1 tsp. ground cumin
1 tsp. ground coriander
1 tsp. curry powder
pinch cayenne
salt and pepper to taste

Combine butter, onion, garlic, ginger, potatoes, green beans, carrots, pea pods, and spices in skillet with small amount of water. Saute about 5 minutes. Add red bell pepper, cabbage, and squash. Saute additional 5 minutes. Serves 2.

Salads

There's nothing like a garden fresh salad! Fresh vegetables are full of vitamins, minerals, and fiber. Whether tossed in a wooden bowl or arranged elegantly on the finest china, these delicious gifts of the earth nourish our bodies and keep us healthy and strong. Here are some suggested ingredients. Choose as many or as few as you like!

Romaine, Butter or Red Leaf
   Lettuce
Alfalfa, Clover, Mung or
   Other Sprouts
Red or White Cabbage
Endive
Spinach
Parsley
Cilantro
Sliced Tomatoes

Sliced Cucumber
Sliced Celery
Grated Carrot
Grated Beets
Red, Yellow or Green Bell
   Peppers
Black or Green Olives
Artichoke Hearts
Garbanzo Beans
Enjoy!

Mayonnaise

¼ cup vinegar
2 eggs or egg substitute
1 tsp. salt
½ tsp. pepper

1 tsp. chopped garlic
2 cups high oleic or cold
   pressed oil (safflower,
   sunflower, canola)

It is helpful, but not essential, if all ingredients are room temperature. Put vinegars, eggs, salt, pepper, and garlic in blender. Blend at low speed for 30 seconds. While blender is still running, slowly pour in the oil. It is helpful to have a rubber spatula handy to help stir mixture at the top. When it solidifies, stop blending. (It will become thin and runny if blended too long.)

Curry Mayonnaise Dressing

Add 1 teaspoon of curry powder to 1 cup of homemade mayonnaise. This can be used as a dressing on salads, as a dip for raw vegetables, and even as a sauce for poultry or fish.

Vinaigrette Dressing

1-⅓ cup flax or high oleic
   safflower oil
¼ cup raw cider vinegar or
   lemon juice

½ tsp. garlic powder
½ tsp. basil
½ tsp. oregano
salt and pepper to taste

Blend all ingredients together and serve over favorite salad.

Cole Slaw

2 cups chopped cabbage
1 cup grated carrots

1 tbs. celery seeds
1 cup mayonnaise

Toss cabbage, carrots, and celery seeds together so that they are equally distributed. Fold in mayonnaise until all ingredients are coated.

Fiesta Kraut

1 cup shredded red cabbage
1 cup grated carrot
1 cup grated beets
¼ cup grated apple (optional)
1 cup whole cranberries
  (optional)
1 tsp. finely minced garlic

1 tsp. finely grated ginger
dash cinnamon
pinch nutmeg
¼ tsp. orange rind
unpasteurized apple cider
  vinegar to taste
salt and pepper to taste

Combine all ingredients in a large bowl and toss well. A delicious, zingy wake up for the taste buds!

Smoothie

*Smoothies are a great way to start the day, or make
great between-meal snacks.*

In blender, combine:
8 oz. Calli Tea (hot or cold)
1 Tbs. Bee Pollen

3 Tbs. NuPlus
1 Tbs. Almond Butter
Sweeten to taste

Smoothie Supreme

In blender, combine:
5 oz. Almond Amazake (not
  for people with yeast
  overgrowth or
  hypoglycemia)
2 Tbs. Bee Pollen

5 oz. Calli and Fortune
  Delight or other herbal tea
1–3 Tbs. NuPlus
½ Tsp. Acidophilus Powder
1 Raw Egg Yolk

Ultimate Smoothie

In blender, combine:
10 oz. water or herb tea
1-3 Tbs. NuPlus
1–3 Quinary Packs
6 Capsules Korean Ginseng*
½ Tsp. Acidophilus Powder

6 Capsules Action Caps*
1 Tbs. Bee Pollen
1-2 tsp. Flax Seed Oil
1 Raw Egg Yolk
Sweeten to taste

*Note: Empty powder from capsules, except Action Cap Formula #1, and blend with other ingredients.

Wizard's Delite

12 oz. Calli Tea
½ tsp. Acidophilus Powder
½ tsp. DL Phenylalanine
¼–½ tsp. Fortune Delight
(optional)
1-2 tsp. Flax Seed Oil

1 tbs. Raw Almond Butter
6 Action Caps #2 & #3
6 Korean Ginseng Capsules
1–3 Quinary Packets
2 Tbs. Bee Pollen
1-3 Tbs. NuPlus

Combine all ingredients in blender. Take this smoothie with 1 Beauty Pearl, Mezotrace, 200 Mg. Vitamin C, and 50 Mg. Coenzyme Q10. Enjoy the lift!

* 3 Action Cap Capsules may be swallowed.

CHAPTER 11

Rebuilding the Co-Dependent

We have no figures for the addiction we call co-dependence. But we are now coming to terms with the overwhelming incidence of this disease. John Bradshaw labels our society "co-dependent-compulsive," full of sexual denial and emotional abuse. He notes that in this country alone, 34 million women are known to have been victims of incest and 10 million people a year are victims of violence from within their family of origin. These are the reported cases. How many hundreds of thousands go unreported?

AA has a dictum: "Addicts don't have relationships: they take hostages." This is a reality of addict/co-dependent liaisons. Many people are incapable of real friendship. They don't want to take responsibility for their own lives. Instead, they find practitioners and "friends" (co-dependents) to take care of them while they continue their self-destructive ways. This is such a vast and pervasive condition—and most of us are so thoroughly immersed in it—that it is difficult even to recognize it let alone know how to change.

The first step in healing co-dependency is to recognize that you are expending tremendous energy helping or trying to "fix" others—while your own life is unmanageable. The second step is to learn to love and care for yourself—*before anyone else.*

171

Perhaps this seems like a prescription for selfishness, but experience is teaching us that we cannot love others unless we first love ourselves. A growing body of self-help books aimed at teaching recovering addicts and co-dependents how to nurture, re-parent, and honor themselves provide testimony to a need to focus on the self first.

Each individual has a duty to care for and be responsible for him or herself. Otherwise we condone and perpetuate a caste society, where some are here only to serve others—with no *personal* responsibility for our own existence and no universal connection. Until we can love and be responsible for the Self, we can only offer band-aid solutions to other people's and the world's problems.

CARETAKING AND WEAK BOUNDARIES

Co-dependents are typically people who feel responsible for the world but cannot take responsibility for their own lives. They give of themselves constantly, but find it extremely difficult, if not impossible, to receive. Co-dependents are experts at taking care of everyone, including the casual acquaintance.

Wanda, a 33-year-old mother, was working two jobs and unable to meet her debts and personal needs. Most of her earnings were used to pay for babysitting for her 2½-year-old son. Her new neighbor, Clara, became sick. Wanda loaned Clara money to pay her rent, even though she barely knew the woman. A few days later, Clara's car broke down so Wanda felt compelled to lend her car, as well. Wanda found herself asking her employer for transportation, or having to take buses, as she was unable to set any limits on Clara's use of her vehicle. Typical of co-dependents, Wanda has no boundaries. Nothing is too much.

Carolyn's 24-year-old son suffered a nervous breakdown. During his recovery in a half-way house, he developed a relationship with a woman. She was ready to move out before he was. He asked Carolyn to pay the rent on his girlfriend's new apartment, as there was "no one else to turn to." Carolyn cried, pleading with her son not to ask such things of her again, but was unable to refuse. She had only met the girlfriend once.

If someone was in need, and Carolyn had the resources, she could not refuse. She felt obliged to give, no matter how difficult it made her own life. She might resent it, and complain bitterly, but saying no was impossible.

OBSESSION AND CONTROL

Co-dependents become obsessed with other people. They focus all their energy on the problems of others. They often have great insights about the addict they relate to, and can talk for hours about how they act, think, feel, and what they should be doing, thinking, feeling. They scrutinize the addict's behavior, always thinking: "If only he/she would do this, or that, they would make my life so much more pleasant, or bearable." They see the "potential" in the addict and keep trying, through control and manipulation, to steer the addict to become a "better person," never able to accept the addict on his own terms. And they feel so justified! What nobler cause than to try to reform an addict?

But co-dependents are unable to see themselves. They don't know what they feel or think, and manage to avoid getting in touch with themselves by constantly being concerned with others' (especially the addict's) problems. They do not act, they simply react.

My own life was totally out of control. Yet I kept thinking that if only my lover would do this and not that, my life would be fine. I could be feeling wonderful, productive, alive. A phone call from him could put me in an emotional downspin that lasted for days. During those times, I felt strung out and nervous; my stomach was in knots. My whole body remained tense and rigid. I made mistakes while driving—often barely escaping serious injury. I had insomnia, coupled with what I call midnight madness where I would fantasize conversations in which I would express all my needs/wants/desires. I was so articulate! I'd plan the next visit and how I would tell him so many things.

And he would understand and all would be well. Or: I would tell him off. We would be finished. I would be free.

I vowed to make changes on our next visit every week. And every week, he would have what I perceived as needs, and I would say to myself: This isn't the time. I'll wait until his situation is better, so he will be receptive. But the time never came. I always saw his needs as greater than mine and was never able to do it. And should we have a fight, I would try to say some of the things I had fantasized and they would come out all wrong and out of context, and only serve to worsen the situation. Somehow I managed to sabotage anything that might serve me.

My behavior was aimed at controlling my lover, his actions, his thoughts and who he was. In relations with other people, I was the same: always trying to influence them, get them to take my advice, my counsel, and do it my way. I often took on the responsibilities of others as I was certain that my way was the only way to do something. This characteristic also would not allow others to do for me, as again, my way was the best, and I always had to impose it on the situation.

THE MARTYR

The martyr syndrome is classic. Co-dependents willingly sacrifice themselves and then complain bitterly because they feel unappreciated. Yet they are so unable to receive that they literally run from anyone who might give to them.

Carolyn said: "It took me years to figure out why I couldn't attract a man into my life who treated me well. As I achieved a little recovery, I noticed that whenever I was around someone who wanted to wait on me (it could be as simple as getting me a glass of water) I got very uncomfortable. I was afraid to be with someone who served me: I needed to be the server. I was comfortable only when I was taking care of the other person, no matter how hard it was (I might even be ill myself). I could always 'rise to the occasion' if the other person had what I perceived as a need. I might even get high on serving (look at what a wonderful person I am) and then feel depressed because 'no one would ever do so much for me.' (Of course I wouldn't let them if they tried.)"

Martyrs feel trapped. It's a catch-22: they are "damned if they do and damned if they don't. " Carolyn's mother felt so helpless and hopeless about her alcoholic husband. Try as she might, she couldn't change him. The more she tried, the more he drank—to avoid her henpecking as well as escape the pressures and responsibilities of his out-of-control life.

CO-DEPENDENTS FEEL MORE ALIVE IN THE MIDST OF A CRISIS

Co-dependents have great difficulty being with themselves. They rush madly from one crisis to the next. Calmness and serenity are too frightening and when things are going smoothly they think it is "too good to be true" and surely to be followed by disaster. And they (unconsciously) create the disaster so they can run to the rescue and be needed, or prove that good things never happen to them. "Murphy's Law" must surely have been written by a co-dependent. The idea that if something can go wrong, it will is the co-dependent's theme song.

VICTIMS

Society validates the co-dependent—the one who will work late, go the extra mile, work the extra shift, clean up the messes and spills, make the phone calls and excuses when the addict can't make it to work, loan (or give) money to almost anybody who asks, and so on ad infinitum. Co-dependents probably keep much of society afloat, never asking for or accepting extra payment for giving far more than is required or expected by a "normal" person. Co-dependence is supported, fostered and encouraged by our culture. Indeed, it is seen as a positive way to function. Co-dependents are willing to do whatever it takes to be liked. Co-dependents often become workaholics, too obsessed with taking care of the world to tend to their own needs.

But mostly, co-dependents are victims. The victims of alcoholism and other compulsive disorders of the people in their lives. Co-dependents desperately need help. They need to learn how to establish and maintain boundaries; to validate and learn to care for themselves, and to stop trying to control others. They need to recognize when their own lives are out of control; and that others' actions dictate their own sense of well-being, indeed, their own sense of self.

Sharon Wegscheider-Cruise, a family therapist and author, has estimated that 96 percent of the U.S. population suffers from co-dependence.

RECOVERY

Recovery from co-dependence is a long and difficult process. In a sense, it is more difficult than recovery from substance abuse. At least not using can be seen as progress.[1] How does the co-dependent begin to stop taking care of others, when that is all she knows how to do? And she has felt so "right," so "correct," so "necessary" for so long.

Recognizing the symptoms is a first step. Co-dependents, like substance abusers, are in denial about their problem. I went reluctantly to a few Al-Anon meetings while still in relationship with an addict. I resented having to go to meetings for *his* problem. I had "more important" things to do with my time— which was filled with running other people's lives.

But observing that I could become an emotional basket case simply because of a comment from my lover or son helped me to be open to getting help. I wanted to develop "detachment" and "unconditional love." These were vague terms to me, but they sounded good and became the focus of my search. I thought there must be something wrong if two of the people I loved most in this world could cause me so much pain. Where was the joy of loving? It seemed I hadn't experienced much of that for years.

With the help of a spiritual program and therapy, I was able to break off my seven-year relationship with an addict (who was two years sober and regularly attending AA). I had been unable to change habitual ways of relating (needing to control, and taking responsibility for his needs and feeling resentful) while still in the relationship.

Later, I got into an Al-Anon ACA program. I remember my first meeting: as each person shared, I was mentally keeping track of their problem. I had a 'fix' plan for every one and would approach them after the meeting. I thought I could be the saviour of all those people! When I told them what to do, all would be well.

Luckily, before the meeting concluded, thanks to the share from 'Helene,' I realized that rescuing was an unhealthy characteristic. I realized that I needed this program if I was ever to find a way to stop.

Recovery requires a multi-faceted approach. There is no one way and each person must find the combination of factors and forces that contribute to the process. Mental, physical, emotional, and spiritual aspects all require attention. A primary factor is the conscious decision to do something about your life. No one can do this for you.

Co-dependents are masters at persistence and constancy. Take a look at how much of these two attributes it has taken to be a co-dependent to other people; how you have stuck to your guns with determination and conviction that you were right and could effect positive change. The task today is to apply these attributes to your own recovery program. But do it lovingly. Don't beat yourself up because you aren't perfect, because you can't do it all today, or this month, or this year.

Self-esteem is at the top of the list. Up until now, you have been unable to give to yourself because you deemed others more worthy than you.

More than two years ago a hypnotherapist took me back to my childhood and I got in touch with my inner child. He asked me to hold her. I couldn't. I didn't like her. No one else had wanted to hold and love her, so why should I? On the mental-emotional level I was shocked and dismayed by this. Who can resist a beautiful, innocent child? But on a feeling level, I had an aversion to connecting with this little girl who had been so invalidated. She was not worth my attention or love.

This new awareness gave me something to work with. I needed to connect with that inner child and begin to accept, then validate, nourish and love her. I looked at the few things I could remember.[2] I noticed that who I was as a child was not validated. I had to be what my parents and siblings wanted me to be. Acceptance and validation were there for "the good girl," "the tap dancer" (if she practiced), the "do as you are told" girl, the "go to bed on time" girl, the "helper."

But the little girl who was afraid of the dark, or of an explosion happening while the dentist's drill was in her mouth, or of our house sliding down into the 100-foot drop behind it—the girl who had fears and a child's perception of the world—was not accepted. It was not okay to be afraid. It was not okay to be disappointed when promises were not kept. I had to be a "big girl." Being a "big girl" meant being responsible, taking care of others and not being a burden to them.

How many of us grew up believing we were "burdens"? We believed we had to make up for it by being perfect and taking care of the rest of the world so as to lessen the "burden," and to make our existence worthwhile, or tolerable, for others.

Developing self-esteem can begin with setting boundaries, defining who you are and what is acceptable to you. A very powerful step can be as simple as unplugging your phone at night, cutting off your 24-hour-a-day availability for crises. Another can be refusing to miss your meeting or class because of another's need.

Get in touch with your inner child and begin to validate and love it. Be patient. It may take a while. I believe that 12-step meetings are invaluable. At nearly every meeting someone will speak of their initial resistance to the meetings and the program, but go on to say how incredibly important they became for their sanity, serenity and ability at times to simply get through the next few hours.

Rebuilding the physical health of the co-dependent follows similar principles and formulas for rebuilding the addict. The strain and lack of self care in your life may have created adrenal and nervous system exhaustion, liver and digestive malfunction, hypoglycemia, and nutritional deficiencies. You can benefit from eating good, regular meals and using strengthening formulas.

Just remember that healing is possible. The road is not easy, but the rewards on the path are great. Serenity and sanity can become normal. You are worth it!

See the chapter entitled "Getting Help" (starting on page 9) for more specifics on body work, emotional support, groups, and other therapies.

Endnotes to Chapter 11

1. This is not meant to denigrate the plight of the addict. Indeed, probably every recovering addict must eventually come to grips with his or her co-dependency. But that is the final addiction, the one that doesn't get attention until the others are well in hand.

2. It is common with traumatized people—and all addicts/co-dependents have been traumatized—that painful memories are blocked. Whole periods of life are beyond recall. At this point, I can remember only one Christmas from my childhood. Drunkenness and dysfunction in my family made all those times too painful to remember.

CHAPTER 12
Case Histories

FREE FROM COCAINE

"I want to relate some of the experiences of my brother Ken. Over a period of three years, Ken developed a serious cocaine habit which eventually sapped all his considerable financial resources. The lifestyle which accompanied his cocaine abuse included hard liquor and a terribly poor diet (all fast food).

"I saw Ken and his family in the summer of 1986. His wife pulled me aside and asked me to keep an eye on him; she feared he was developing muscular dystrophy. He had so succeeded in cloaking his habit that his wife was aware only of the inevitable symptoms of abuse. Ken's fists were constantly clenched and his facial muscles were often contorted in an ugly manner. He was very fidgety and nervous (actually paranoid).

"The three months that followed were very bad ones for Ken and his family. Things went from bad to worse and he finally hit rock bottom.

"Through a friend with a similar problem, my brother found out about some herbal formulas. While these products were not marketed with any claims of curing substance abuse, they nonetheless helped him immensely. He started drinking copious amounts of two cleansing teas (Calli and Fortune Delight), using

181

NuPlus, Prime Again, Alpha 20C and weight-loss formulas. He lost weight quickly (30 pounds) and his whole outlook on life underwent an incredible metamorphosis. He told me that his cravings for cocaine, liquor and even cola soft drinks suddenly came to an end. Whole foods suddenly tasted good to him, and he had the energy to tackle new, demanding work.

"He went out and got the first job he had held in years. He started doing heavy labor at a construction site, and through using the formulas he surprised everyone, including himself, by being able to maintain the very demanding pace. This was especially remarkable as even for years before using cocaine, he had been overweight and living a lazy life on colas, coffee and pizza.

"Ken's family and friends were totally amazed at the changes in him. He became a responsive, caring parent and husband.

"My brother credits the herbs with his recovery and he is well aware that he has to continue using them in an ongoing mainte-nance program. Whenever he has temporarily run out of the herbs, he has noticed himself backsliding—not to cocaine, but to beer, soft drinks and junk food. After a few such episodes, he has come to see how essential the formulas are in maintaining a proper balance in his body.

"I relate this not to convince people to try to treat themselves for problems with addiction. For instance, counselling seems to be an important component in any treatment program, but is something my brother wholly neglected. Perhaps Ken was just incredibly lucky (although I'm not sure I believe in luck) and discovered formulas which were perfectly attuned to his physi-cal need at that point in time. At any rate, I am grateful as a loving brother for the wonderful outcome."

HALCION MADNESS

"After several months of Chronic Fatigue Syndrome (commonly called Epstein-Barr Virus), suffering from various flu-like symp-toms, and becoming debilitated to the point of being almost totally bedridden, I began to have more and more difficulty falling asleep and staying asleep. A night of interrupted sleep or just a few hours of sleep left me devastatingly exhausted and ill for the next day or even for several days.

"My doctor prescribed a commonly-used sleeping pill called Halcion. I usually was very wary of drugs and their side effects, but I was desperate and he assured me this was a very mild, yet effective, non-addictive sleeping pill. Peaceful dreams were mine at last. I fell asleep quickly and easily and slept restfully for a full eight hours.

"Over the next year, I noticed I needed larger and more frequent doses of Halcion to get the same effect. I didn't dare think about trying to sleep without it. I was still too sick with CFS to think of enduring any sleepless nights. I thought I'd wait until I was well again, then deal with the sleeping pill issue, which seemed small compared to my illness.

"I started noticing increasing feelings of confusion, irritability and depression. I met another doctor, and we became friends. One day he told me he suspected I was addicted to Halcion. I was shocked. How could this be? My regular doctor had told me repeatedly that Halcion is a safe medication and I had believed him. (Today I would say I don't think there is such a thing as a safe drug.)

"My doctor friend continued to describe side effects of the drug, and I fit the picture. Now I knew I had to get off Halcion. To my dismay I found I simply could not do without it. Withdrawal was sheer living hell. For months, I struggled with different programs. But even Valium couldn't get me through the withdrawal. My body craved Halcion even more. If I did not take Halcion every six hours, I experienced tortuous withdrawal symptoms. By this time I was experiencing memory loss and intense suicidal feelings, added to the depression and confusion I was already experiencing. I called a detox center, but they wouldn't take me because I was still so sick with the CFS.

"Meanwhile, I started a new herbal nutritional program, which was highly recommended by a friend. After a few weeks, I decided to try again to stop using Halcion. I was going crazy and my life was hardly endurable. Suicide was a daily consideration.

"A friend of mine who had previously been addicted to Halcion and knew how much I was suffering gave me three or four of his mild tranquilizers. (I had given up on any of my doctors' programs, as none of them had worked.) I was totally off Halcion in three days. I took a tranquilizer once or twice, then never again. I was taking herbal formulas four or five times a day, especially the three formulas for the nervous system. I hardly went through any withdrawal at all. It was like a miracle. It was so easy, I could hardly believe it.

"I've never taken Halcion since nor experienced any great difficulty sleeping. Some nights I take extra herbal nervous system formulas to relax me and help me sleep more deeply.

"I have done a lot of research on Halcion since then, and have found it is illegal in many European countries due to its link to suicides. I have heard of and met many people who have experienced the Halcion hell. This drug is a nightmare for many and even the cause of death for some.

"I am grateful to the nutritional program, which I believe so boosted and nourished my body that I could get free without the agony of withdrawal."

A 28-DAY MIRACLE

"I remember having my first glass of wine—at my grandparents' house—and how good it felt. I always wanted to go back to their house to drink that glass of wine. And then it became two or three glasses of wine. I really enjoyed the effect of it.

"I have always been a heavy-set person, and when I was 12, Mom took me to a doctor to lose some weight. That doctor prescribed dexedrine, two every morning, noon and night. So at 12 I was using amphetamines and drinking on a regular basis.

"I come from a family of substance abusers, though none of us thought of ourselves as substance abusers. My father was a very heavy drinker and Mom is into pharmaceuticals. Seven years ago, we had to rush her to the hospital. She was taking between 500 and 1000 codeine pills a month, but couldn't understand why her stomach closed up.

"Growing up as a child was a pleasant experience and a not-so-pleasant experience. My dad had a real mean streak when he was drinking, which was most of the time. There was a lot of love, but when Dad was drinking, you just wanted to stay out of his way. Mealtime at our house was not a real happy time. Mother didn't sit at the table, because if Dad didn't like what he had to eat, my mom got to wear it. She would pull out a little bread board in the kitchen and put her plate there, and most of the time she sat away from the table so as not to deal with that.

"There was always bottle of Johnny Walker Red label at one end of the table and a bottle of Jim Beam at the other end, and we all had a shot of booze before dinner. There was never anything said about booze being bad or anything like that.

"I was a loner most of my life—a heavy-set kid with a bunch of pimples on my face—so I didn't mix in with the other kids. I stayed home; I had a stamp collection and did things by myself. When I was about 14, I had to go to the hospital to have my stomach pumped. I went into alcoholic shock after drinking nearly a quart of scotch. I was quite sick, and the doctors feared I might die.

"At 18 I was drinking a case of beer a day and still taking amphetamines, but the dose had increased to six three times a day, instead of two.

"I never thought there was anything wrong with drinking. Hanging out at bars and drinking was normal. I knew nothing else. And I always worked with guys that drank a lot. I hung out with drinkers. Yeah, I got drunk, I had hangovers, but my dad did the same thing. The different bosses I had were all heavy drinkers. I started having business lunches that would include three or four drinks.

"I married twice, and I met both my wives at bars. I was abusive with my first wife. She needled me a lot, and so I punched her in the arm. That marriage was filled with a lot of yelling and screaming—plenty of verbal abuse. The nicest thing to come from the marriage is my son. He is 21.

"I had stayed away from other drugs because my brother was a heroin junkie and I didn't like that. But I took a lady home from a bar one night and she talked me into smoking a joint. I passed out on her couch and woke up next morning with a terrible hangover. She talked me into another joint and it took my headache away. That started my addiction to marijuana.

"Then I was at a party one night and a mirror came around and I said no, I don't do that. Then the mirror came around the second time and before you know it, I put that white powder in my nose and cocaine was my next love.

"Whatever it was, if it was a substance that made you feel different, I used it. I didn't get paranoid from using. I didn't use because I was lonely. I didn't use to escape from anything. I used because I liked to get loaded and the more loaded I got the better I liked it and the fact that I could use cocaine and prolong my use was that much better because I didn't like to fall asleep too early. Then someone gave me speed. I started out using six a day.

"It was during my second marriage, after a lot of years of using and abusing—I don't know where I crossed that line, whatever that imaginary line is—but I became victim of that king alcohol and then I had no choice whether I wanted to drink or not. I lost track of when I took my first drink in the morning—I don't even remember that.

"I have this large glass coffee table—about 3½ feet square—and I would run a line of cocaine all the way around that table. And I would sit in my chair drinking, and I would get up and do one side with one nostril and then the other . . .

"I had a lot of paraphernalia and became quite a connoisseur. I had the finest of the fine. That was the love of my life. I wasn't in love with any particular person. I was in love with all of the drugs. I loved to take care of them. I had special places to keep them, special jars. I'm an obsessive-compulsive person so when I got a little low on anything, I had to go out and buy a quantity of it. I never bought a lid of weed, I bought it by the half pound or quarter pound. I rolled up 40 or 50 joints at a time. The whole thing got away from me.

"Every Saturday I'd buy the same thing: two half gallons of vodka, six half gallons of white wine, and two liters of Korbel Brandy. That is the booze I drank from Saturday to Saturday.

"I had quit drinking scotch because I had a problem with hemorrhoids and the doctor told me I had to drink white wine or vodka. So I basically listened to my doctor.

"I belong to a men's club and I went there for lunch every day. I used to beat the crowd by about 15 minutes because my hands were shaking so bad I couldn't lift up a glass. I got behind the bar and poured myself a whole glass of booze and put my face down to the glass and lifted it up so I could down it quick and the shakes would quit by the time the rest of the men got there.

"When I woke up in the morning I had the shakes so bad it was all I could do to get into the bathroom and grab my bottle of blues (10 mg. Valium). I would take two blues and down that with vodka. Then pretty soon I would be on my hands and knees throwing up. I had to get rid of it. You know, that virgin stomach, when the booze goes down the first thing. All alcoholics wind up the same way. And I would throw up blood at the same time. The blood bothered me at first and I went to the doctor. He told me I had diverticulitis and gave me Tagamet. Then he gave me Valium for what he called a nervous condition and upset stomach. That started me on the blues.

"Then while my wife was in the shower, I would get the vodka out of the refrigerator and drink right out of the bottle. As soon as she left for work, I'd grab the wine, because even with the Valiums I was still shaking and I had to have some wine and I was sure I needed something with a lot of sugar in it.

"When I left for work every morning, I was a walking time-bomb. I carried a little brass tin with nine or 10 joints in my right hand rear pocket, and in my left hand front pocket was an empty cocaine bottle and in my right front pocket was a full bottle—you know those little coke bottles with a spoon—and in my inside coat pocket was a flask full of vodka. I also carried a pill box full of blues. Then at work, while others had coffee in their cups, I had booze in mine. I had a private bathroom off my office and I would go in there and light up a joint.

"That is the way I spent my life. I'd go to my men's club for lunch. I'd get through lunch and the shakes would start and then pains in my chest and I was afraid I was having a heart attack.

There was only one way to get rid of that feeling. Eight to 10 or 12 ounces of brandy (and later, vodka) got rid of the pains and I was good for another couple of hours.

"I never went to sleep at night, I just passed out. At 42 or 43 (I'm now 49), when I got home from work I'd pour another big fat drink, fire up a joint and sit in my favorite chair and pass out. And maybe if I woke up at two in the morning I'd get into bed and sometimes I wouldn't wake up at all. I'd come to at three or four in the morning and take a shower and have that drink and the insanity would start all over again.

"In the last year of my drinking I wasn't eating any food at all. All I was doing was drinking. I was one sick human being. I weighed 245 pounds and I was sick. I sweat at night. My wife couldn't sleep with me.

"On January 24, 1985, I woke up and couldn't get out of bed. I couldn't move my legs. I was paralyzed from my waist down. I knew I had to get to the bathroom because I was shaking and needed a drink. I rolled off the bed and dragged myself into the bathroom and it was all I could do to grab my blues, and my bottle of booze I kept in there. Nothing would stay down. I was laying in my own vomit and I was through yelling for God to help me. I said could somebody please help me.

"My wife got me to the hospital. I wound up with the DT's. I had pneumonia. My kidneys weren't functioning at all. My liver was off the chart. I was no better, no worse than any junkie, any alcoholic that winds up on the curb. The only thing was that I had a house to live in, otherwise, I would be laying in the curb. I wasn't broke, I still had some money in my pocket.

"I had a room next to intensive care so the nurses could watch me. A woman came and told me she was alcoholic, and shared her story. She held me all day. The doctor said I might make it. If I got beyond 10 days, I might have a chance, he said, and suggested I get into a program. I smelled bad, looked bad, my hygiene was poor—I was real sick.

"A couple of ladies came to visit me from MPI (Merritt Peralta Institute) and suggested I go through the 28-day program. The next day they came with a form for me to sign. I'll never forget that day. My hands were shaking so bad that I signed my name with an x. In the Big Book of AA they talk about the 'pitiful and incomprehensible demoralization' and that is exactly where I was. That day I was able to push myself around the room with an aluminum walker. On my seventh day I checked into MPI. Jan. 31, 1985. Since that time I haven't found the need to use or drink anything. I've been clean ever since.

"I remember Jean, my therapist. I hated her the month I was at MPI but now I worship the ground she walks on. She has a job I wouldn't want to have. Then there is the director: Rich Pelletier. Those people saw I was a human being and had a lot of empathy and compassion and they helped me get through that month.

"Many times I thought they were trying to break me down emotionally and physically and get me to do something that was not natural for me. I was scared to death. Today I see it was a comprehensive program of understanding about the disease of alcoholism and understanding myself.

"Some of the meetings I went to have been lasting. We started dealing with feelings. I had been to psychologists and psychiatrists before but nobody dealt with the things they dealt with. What I really like about MPI is that all the people that run the place are former users. So I was dealing with people who really understood where I came from and the feelings I had and why I drank and used the way I did. They could share that experience and strength and instill the hope in me that they recovered and I could to.

"I came away from that 28 days with two years worth of knowledge. Had I just gone into AA and NA off the street, it would have taken me at least two years, maybe three, to gain the knowledge I got there in 28 days. I sponsor a guy now that has been in program 2½ years and he is just at the point that people are after just 28 days at MPI.

"They had special assignments. I didn't understand it at the time. I had to write all the pay-offs and negative consequences of being a polyanna. List at least 10 different things. I said I wasn't a polyanna but Jean said do it anyway. I have all the stuff from the program in a folder by my bed and every now and again I look at it.

"Today I am active in AA and NA, I sponsor a few guys and go to eight or nine meetings a week. Not because I have to, I want to. I never really had a Higher Power in my life but I do today. I don't know if I believe it all but my favorite cliche is "fake it till you make it." I learned that at the beginning of my recovery. I was having a problem with my Third Step and this guy told me whether you believe this stuff or not, just make believe you believe it. That is the way I worked a lot of this program. I faked it till I believed it. But I have no fear of the program, nobody has ever hurt me.

"I also volunteer at MPI and so I get to meet 400 to 500 people a year that go thru that place and I think more people do recover than don't. They have tremendous after care. A one-year program that you pay for at the beginning. But I know people who went through that aftercare with me five years ago and I'm sure they don't pay anything extra to stay in it.

"One person said it is a "We" program—we do it together. And that is one of the things that has really helped me. There is a way today. You just have to be willing to change your entire life—have to be willing to change. If it worked for me, it can work for anybody. I was a hope-to-die-drunk and a hope-to-die-drug-fiend and there was no way in the world I could stop. It is a miracle. It is by God's grace that I don't have to drink and use anymore. I do the footwork.

"I was impotent for nearly three years after getting sober. I was going out with a woman and so she took me to a chiropractor/nutritionist and he started me on a whole new eating regime with a properly balanced diet, and complex carbohydrates and lots of vitamin supplements. And I saw an acupuncturist—actually an OMD (Oriental Medical Doctor).

"It took me a long time to start feeling good—but it started after that. I didn't know what it was like to be sober. I hadn't been sober since I was a kid. I had met one guy who started feeling good in about six months. The way I felt bad was I was light-headed and dizzy all the time. I didn't know if it would ever go away.

"My only problem today is I like to eat too much. The only side effect is that I sometimes get anxiety—the residual of Valium. I may never overcome that. A friend with 14 years' sobriety has the same symptoms. It is important to talk to others. It helps to know that you aren't the only one.

"I used to take Maxide for my heart and Lasix because I couldn't urinate. I was told I would have to take these pills for the rest of my life because of the damage I had done to my liver, kidneys and heart. But I weaned myself off of these after I started eating properly and taking herbs the acupuncturist gave me. I did it with just nutrition. Today I don't take anything except vitamins and six to seven grams of vitamin C.

"About three years ago MPI did a pilot "step-ahead" program. I was one of six picked to go through it. Four men, two women. We were together from 6 a.m. till 11:30 p.m. daily. It was focused on life beyond recovery. You need two years' recovery to qualify. So I got to work a week with Tim Cermack, a Psychiatrist who is also national director and founder of Adult Children of Alcoholics. That one week took my recovery a long way. I was able to deal with my father. I had never dealt with him before. I got some freedom from some of the bad feelings I had.

"I am such a fortunate human being to have become an alcoholic and drug addict. How the hell else would I have found what I have today? I wouldn't have this without that program. I believe there is a reason for everything happening in life. It was meant to be. It is great!"

RUNNING SCARED

"I started doing drugs in the 1960s. I used pot, amphetamines and LSD, then progressed—like most of the kids in the neighborhood—to heroin, which I did for 12 to 13 years. During that time I was on two methadone programs.

"My upbringing was nothing traumatic, but when I got into treatment I started to look at it. My Irish father was not very affectionate or emotional. And my mother was overprotective, she didn't give me the freedom to go out and explore and be with the guys and to simply grow up. I realize now that there was emotional abuse. Growing up is difficult enough, kids are insecure beings. But my father started calling me a lot of bad names and that I could not understand. I didn't start doing drugs then, but I certainly was growing up not feeling very good about myself, not feeling very confident.

"I went to Catholic schools. In High School I ran track and cross-country and was always involved in sports. I was a very good athlete and didn't drink or do drugs.

"But when it was time to get ready for college, time to develop a social life, to date, and do all the things that guys do, I didn't have the confidence or security to do it. What I found gave me that confidence, what made me feel good, was chemical, a substance, a drug. Amphetamines did that. They made me feel on top of the world. I took barbiturates and I didn't have any problems. When I went to clubs and I had to talk to a woman, I found a chemical gave me the confidence. And it gave me the confidence to hang out and be one of the guys. I turned to drugs to make me feel better about myself.

"I was given material things many kids don't have. I had a good home, my father didn't give me emotional support, but he was there. He worked a lot, fourteen, sixteen, eighteen hours a day. He drank only the occasional beer.

"Once I started shooting heroin, everything went down hill. I was used to a warm bed and a nice place to live. And I found myself in shooting galleries, in abandoned buildings, walking around Manhattan going to blood banks to get money for food or drugs, sleeping on park benches. In an abandoned building, I was tapping into water pipes to get water for heroin and to get high.

"My drug use got worse. I got arrested, found myself in jail, eventually in a detox ward at St. Luke's Hospital in New York—which is a locked facility. I was taking methadone and I was very sick. Although the withdrawal and the whole experience was very bad, when I left the hospital I went back to drugs. When I quit I was doing $200 heroin a day. As much drugs I could get, that was how much I would do.

"But there came a time when the drugs no longer worked for me, didn't give me that confidence and security anymore. I was kind of down on life and wishing I had the courage to kill myself. Towards the end I withdrew from the world, I wouldn't answer the phone. The only thing I did was go out to get money, get high and be alone, get more drugs and come home and be alone again.

"I had tried to kick drugs many times, just went cold turkey for a lot of years and every time I would clean up, I would go back. I never stopped. It is kind of funny, when I started to stop is when I had money. Living in a big house, car parked out front. But it wasn't fun anymore. I was very unhappy, lonely, depressed, wishing I was dead. Although I had material things, I didn't have friends.

"Money wasn't a problem, I had an inheritance. Although earlier on, it was. I stole from family and friends and would try to steal cars, and all that.

"My family didn't know what to do with me. My parents were no longer living, but my sister and my uncles tried to get through to me.

"I reached a point where I just wanted to die. I didn't know what to do. Coming home from a methadone program one day, sitting and waiting for the F train, a guy sat down next to me and asked me what I was doing. I told him about the methadone program and he told me I could clean my life up and he gave me the Daytop Village phone number.

"I had no intention of calling but when I got home my sister was there and I mentioned the experience. She made a phone call and set up an interview for me. Their recommendation was that I needed a therapeutic community which is long term, I needed a live-in program. But I was not ready to make that commitment. I was afraid, so I decided to shoot dope again.

"Toward the end it got very bad. Drugs didn't mean anything, living didn't mean anything, family didn't mean anything. I certainly didn't care about myself. I was hanging out with the down and out people, the bums, the derelicts. I was about 28. I came into treatment at 29.

"Even though I was shooting, this Daytop thing stuck somewhere in the back of my mind. One day I was with these bums, and I shot $200 worth of dope and it didn't do it. I just wanted to die. Above my head there was a phone on the wall, I'll never forget. I called my sister and said Kathy I can't do this anymore, I need help and she called Daytop Village. The next day they took me in. June 18, 1979. I am clean nearly 11 years now. I don't do caffeine, I don't smoke.

"Daytop is an amazing place. I really thought I'd be a dope fiend the rest of my life. I was never able to stop, after 13 years. But here I am at Daytop Village, with all these people who are ex-drug addicts and I'm looking around and they are just like me. I wanted to leave a lot of times, and do drugs. What kept me there was I started to make friends. People would come over to me and say we care about you, what do you mean you want to leave and they would talk to me and people eventually started telling me they loved me. And I look around and I see people drug free six months, nine months and a year or two and people who had been clean four and five years would come back to the community and visit and do seminars and tell their stories. The individual stories might have been different, but the feelings, what drugs did to their lives were no different.

"Up until about 10½ months I didn't think I would make it. In the back of my mind I thought I'm gonna be a dope fiend all my life. But I stuck it out. I committed myself to the program, to the changes, to what the Daytop concept is: to learn to be honest, to take responsibility for my actions and grow up emotionally.

"I remember waking up one day and it hit me. I thought: maybe, just maybe, I'm not going to shoot dope again. It was like a revelation. Just maybe I'm not going to do drugs. On top of that I had some really good friends. I started to believe in myself again, I started to like who I was becoming, I had the respect of other people. I was getting my own respect back. And I wanted more. I started feeling good and I wanted more. I started having contact with my family again.

"What makes it for me, why I think I am drug and alcohol free now: I live my life by what I learned in Daytop 10½ yrs ago. I learned the way I have to live my life. I don't cheat people, I don't steal or bother people, I try to give back to other kids and adults what I got. I try to help other addicts get it together.

"There is no guarantee I'll spend the rest of my life drug free but certainly I believe my guarantee to stay drug free is to live the concept I learned at Daytop. For me it is to continue living that. Honesty, responsibility, and loving people. Our philosophy is like an affirmation. We say it every day. So we learn new ways of living. I don't hang out with people who do drugs, or in bars. I work for everything I have. I work for it.

"Going through Daytop was the hardest thing I ever did. I wasn't used to being honest. I wasn't used to being responsible, to caring about people, or being open or honest with what I felt. I was used to running, running, running, with drugs. All of a sudden I am in the program at Daytop and I have no drugs, no alcohol too hide behind and I had to face myself. And I faced myself.

"To people who are using: If you want to make it, you can. No one is hopeless. I worked with a man who did drugs 25 years and he is now free.

"To parents I'd like to say: It is not just the person doing drugs: it is a family problem. But there is hope, for the parents, and for the kids. Daytop Village has a family association which helps you get things together.

"One thing I had to learn: a lot of people come into program and they blame. They blame society, their parents, lack of love. They say it was the judge's fault, the probation officer, the social worker's fault—everyone's fault but their own. That is the victim mentality. That is nonsense. I don't blame anyone. I take responsibility for my decision to do dope. The fact my father didn't give me what I needed didn't make me do dope. Yeah, he could have given me more. He made mistakes, but he did the best he could. My decision to do drugs was mine. It was my way of coping, a way of running away. People with that mentality will never get it together. When you get to the point where you take responsibility for that decision then recovery is possible."

MICHAEL

"From the time I was born I was sick between four and six months of every year. I had bronchitis, pneumonia, whooping cough and scarlet fever as well as the whole range of childhood illnesses. I was never well for any length of time.

"At 20, I had a serious physical breakdown. Neither I nor the doctors knew the cause. I was incapacitated for 14 weeks, never really got my energy back, and a few years later developed severe hypoglycemia and a lot of other deteriorating symptoms—problems with my endocrine system, thyroid, adrenals, liver, pancreas, colon, heart and lungs. I relied on laxatives or mechanical means for elimination. My small intestine was not assimilating food and my stomach digestion was faulty. Gas cramps were severe. I had bleeding ulcers and constant nausea from liver and gall bladder malfunction. My pancreas had abscesses and my blood pressure remained dangerously low while my cholesterol and triglycerides were extremely high. My doctors, at first concerned, were now alarmed.

"At that point, I started making significant changes in my diet. I realized I was addicted to sweets. Initially I dealt with it through diet, supplementation and exercise. A few years later, I found a good homeopath and made very definite progress using that method. Herbs were also very helpful. During the whole process, I came to understand a more holistic aspect to health. It took me about seven years to really overcome my sugar craving. It took me much longer than that—11 years—to actually restore my health.

"It took time to understand the emotional component of my heart. I had an addictive personality. My addiction was sugar. Genetically, I could have been predisposed to an addictive type of personality. There was alcoholism two generations back, and my father was a diabetic. The compulsiveness, the obsessive-ness, the going to extremes were there. The addictive part of my personality consistently sabotaged my health care program. I tended to approach my own therapy with the same kind of extremism that I had approached my life. The result was that I traumatized my body and my progress was much slower.

"I began to read about the addictive and co-dependent personality. I sought out support groups from time to time. I got counselling to get the information that would enable me to change, because as long as I had the patterns of emotional imbalance, there was a continuing illness. These imbalances created stress, which created physiological and biochemical imbalances, which eventually created the system of disease in my body.

"For years I had a sarcastic, cynical attitude towards life, and it never occurred to me that that attitude was involved with my illness. The illness sapped my energy. I was so depleted I could not give. I could only take. I was barely surviving and it was too hard to be kind and selfless. Giving up those attitudes was very frightening because I thought it meant giving up my identity. But I found that whenever I faced something and truly met my real needs, there was always something or someone to help. Initially, I thought it was just coincidence. But it has happened so many times, probably hundreds of times over the last 14 years or so, that I've come to trust that process. When I am really ready, the information, individual or book is there for me.

"Over the years I saw that what was required from me was a tremendously steady effort, a sense of hopefulness and humor, and an ability to appreciate each improvement. It was a hard climb to achieve health, but by focusing on just one step at a time, I felt I could do it. If I had tried to look at the whole journey, it would have been overwhelming. By making whatever effort I could, things just seemed to fall into place, and tremendous progress actually happened. It seemed slow at the time, because it took me from 1974 to 1985. Since then I have continued to work on my health. It is excellent now, but I would like it to be magnificent. As my energy has picked up, I have been able to do more of the things that I enjoy. I'm less subject to the stresses in my environment. I enjoy people more.

"Anyone with an addictive nature requires complete support—individual support, informational support, personal support, nutritional support—anything that will work. The journey may be hard, but it's worth it. The effort requires courage and perseverance. It requires gut effort, hope and discrimination. Yet every step we take towards balance, every step we take towards harmony, every time we recognize an extreme for what it is—an aberration—instead of the intense excitement that we think it provides us, moves us into a whole new perspective on life.

"As I have become healthier mentally, emotionally and physically, my energy has increased, and I have found that life is not really the difficult, teacherous process that I had come to think it is. Life is an extremely beautiful process requiring a lot of energy, awareness, focus, and self-knowledge."

"PATRICK"

When I first met Patrick, he was going through his tenth cycle of recovery, success, and relapse. Most of his friends and associates had given up on him by then, and treated him like something rotten than the cat had dragged in. I always experienced a certain wry humor around his escapades, though, and was sure that he would eventually clean up his act and do quite well in life.

There were several years when I never knew whether he was going to pull up to my place in a brand new BMW as the president of some mainline corporation, or if I would be awakened by groans in the middle of the night, walk out onto my porch and stumble over this drunken, ragged, filthy wine-soaked tramp who had crawled away from a month-long binge through the city gutters, stolen and sold everything he could get his hands on, and collapsed on my front deck to hustle some change for one last bottle of rot gut vino.

"Hey, Finn, this life is incredible, huh? He always had the most positive things to say and would often quote scriptures to me in the midst of his debauchery.

"I need a few bucks so I can get some coffee, take the bus down to the detox center and get cleaned up." Bus fare. Right. I was hip to his routine.

"Sure, Patrick. Here, let me make you something to eat, and I just happen to have some bus tokens on hand."

At the mention of bus tokens, his eyes would glaze over like he was ready to kill, and he would mumble , "I'm not really hungry. See you soon, man," take the bus tokens and leave.

Years later, we really laughed over that bus token routine. He went down about as far as a man can go during some of those periods. One time he called me from the hospital after he had been in a coma for three days. They had pumped his stomach and given him transfusions after he was found lying unconscious in an alley, his throat cut and right arm broken. No sooner did I pick up the phone than he began to sing the glory of some great spiritual master or other and recite a few poems of Kabir.

That was Patrick. Just a month before that episode, he had taken me out to dinner at the finest restaurant in town, paid for by his expense account as the head of some nationwide insurance company. We laughed until we cried, and then laughed some more at the wonders of life and love in the midst of material madness. Each moment that we could seize to enjoy our love of life and savor the freeness of our hearts was a moment to be treasured.

When Patrick got out of the hospital, I set him up with some vitamins, herbs, and a nutritional program to help heal his metabolism, loaned him some clothes, and off he went. Two months later, he was president and CEO of another insurance company.

One of the source conflicts and patterns of Patrick's difficulties was that when he started working for a company, he would become very compulsive and get caught up in the momentum of achievement and success. It wouldn't be long after beginning a new job when he would become so concerned with living up to the expectations and demands of his superiors and society, that he would start working long hours, skipping meals, using coffee, Cokes, and sugar to keep going, and not taking time to enjoy the peace and beauty of his life.

I could see it coming and would warn him, "Patrick, you've got to live at a reasonable pace, take time to experience and enjoy your life, and you've got to eat well and use herbs and vitamins to strengthen your metabolism. Your glands and liver function are depleted from years of alcohol and drug abuse, and you have hypoglycemia. If you drive yourself like this you will burn out, crack up, and start drinking again."

He would understand and begin using the nutritional program and take time for himself for a week or two; but then the pressures would build, he would lose control, and after a few months in a driven work environment he would be drinking again.

As soon as he took one drink, that was it. Bye-bye, Baby. Something in his metabolism would go completely insane, and he would down everything he could get his hands on, until he passed out in a drunken stupor. Once a drink passed his lips, his body chemistry would go so haywire that he really had no control over his actions.

His next binge caused a real outcry. He was at his sister's wedding reception, and all his relatives and their friends were there. It was a very formal affair. Patrick was really fried from having driven himself at his job for the previous few months. The stuffy social atmosphere stirred up his rebellion against what he felt was exploitative, materialist nonsense that he wanted nothing to do with. He said screw it, started hitting the champagne, and created a major disturbance. He left town later that night.

There was a big festival coming up in Miami, so Patrick spent every cent he had on a one-way bus ticket, bought six bottles of heavy booze, boarded the bus, and rode to Miami "in style."

You can imagine his condition by the time he arrived. Broke, as well. He slept in vacant lots with refugees and lived on coconuts until I arrived a few days later. By this time he had sold and been robbed of everything he was wearing, except a swimsuit. It was the middle of July, so he was sunburnt badly.

I was staying at the Hilton with some friends and I brought Patrick over to eat and stay with us until the festival was over. Of course, he was drunk the whole time, but at least I could feed him something, lend him some clothes, and put sunburn lotion on him. To me, friendship is sacred, and I couldn't just let him go hungry on the streets.

Patrick stayed on in Miami for a few months, and got a job gardening, while I went back to California. When he returned, he went to work in a nursery and commenced getting his life back together.

I fell into financial hard times, and moved into a cabin in a pecan grove in New Mexico to recover from years of burnout and hard work. I was having a great time playing with the squirrels, writing children's books and telling stories to the kids who came by to visit me.

That was the setting for Patrick's last binge, and it was a doozy. He called saying that he was stressed out, worked to death, and tired of the rat race and trying to live up to everyone's expectations. He wanted to know if he could come to breathe the mellow country air and take some time to appreciate the beauty and love in living. He arrived in El Paso, and I drove down to pick him up with a friend, only to discover that he was totally drunk. I should have known.

We drove back to the cabin, and Patrick and I went for a walk out in the country. A glorious violet sunset streaked the sky, enshrouding the dusky desert mountains that rose in the distance. We hiked through sagebrush and cactus, along a winding stream, talking, trying to find a way to live a life where we could be free and true to the spirit of love that we believed in.

Patrick wandered the town all that night trying to find a liquor store or a bar that was open, then flew back to California the next day, and turned himself over to a detox center.

He straightened out and began working much more closely with the AA twelve step program, which he continues to find invaluable in maintaining his sanity and sobriety. He has developed close friendships with his sponsor and other fellow members who give him a great deal of support, direction, and self-validation.

It's been five years since Patrick's last binge. He is doing quite well now, as president of another big company. He's learning to stay human, continue working with AA, stick with his nutritional program, and enjoy his life, even in the midst of success.

MARY'S STORY

It is frequently suggested that the addict is typically a very sensitive person; an individual who inwardly seeks union with God and who simply cannot bear the separation. Hence the drowning of feelings, the numbing of sensation, the dulling of the mind.

The experience of "Mary," a recovering alcoholic, may serve to illustrate. Mary was hospitalized for a tubal ligation. Fearing that receiving drugs might spiral her back into using, she wanted the smallest amount necessary. So she was given a local, rather than a general, anaesthetic. Following the surgery:

"I was in that twilight zone: not fully conscious, but not totally 'out,' either. An incredibly wonderful vision came to me. I saw beautiful beings, angels of love and light. They said that I had used alcohol and drugs because I wanted to meet with them so much, and that I would do anything to receive them, and experience them. But they told me—they were very loving, and so understanding, so beautiful—that I must not allow myself to use drugs to reach out to them, to try and touch them; they said that I must go through ordinary reality, that going numb to relieve the separation would only delay my journey.

"That happened in the early days of my recovery. I am certain that had I continued to get high, I would not have been able to walk the spiritual path I have been on for the past 10 years. It would have been closed to me. I had to do it the disciplined way. The ego is always in a hurry; it wants to get there quick and easy. But the spiritual path is not quick and easy. We have to go one day at a time.

"That was my first instruction on the path: 'Don't do it that way,' it doesn't work.

"Getting sober and onto my spiritual path was easier after that experience. As I move along my spiritual path, as I am able to remain open and trusting, I continue to receive guidance. And I am forever grateful."

CHAPTER 13

Conclusion

We have offered a survey of information and resources in these pages. Our experience and research led us to these ideas and we present them with humility—in the hope that others may benefit. Your task is to sort out and utilize the parts that fit for you. Each person is an individual—totally unique— while at the same time sharing the human condition with all mankind. Thus, some of our ideas may apply universally while others may be applicable to only a few individuals.

It is our hope that our efforts may contribute to a more widespread understanding of the metabolic—as well as socio-cultural and spiritual—nature of the addictive process and a renewed faith in the possibility of recovery. We have tried to clarify some of the misinformation regarding addiction and co-dependency, realizing also that we cannot possibly cover everything. But pray that this has been comprehensive enough to give most people the understanding and impetus to embark upon their own road to freedom.

Through our study, research, and observation, we perceive that humankind is on the verge of a leap forward. We are not alone in our observation: many attribute the movement toward self actualization to planetary changes and the coming of a "New Age,"[1] others to a resurgence of old values and systems. One author wrote: "This is a time of transcendence." It matters not what we call it. Suffice it to say that significant changes are occurring on our planet which are leading to profound differences in the way people live, communicate and relate.

Many are beginning to regard the disarray, despair, denial, confusion and general hopelessness characterized by these times as opportunity. History teaches us that great changes are imminent when old ways begin to falter and no longer work.[2] People are beginning to believe—and thus demand—that the unfolding of life should offer more, rather than less. Creation is something we all participate in—whether we are conscious of it or not. We are beginning to see beyond the "fall," and affirm that with consciousness comes the desire and ability to change.

A large number of those demanding more of life today are, strangely enough, addicts and co-dependents. A grass-roots movement is developing among the recovery-minded, along with other spiritually oriented individuals and groups. Great efforts are being made to achieve balance. Accepting personal responsibility for oneself is a part of that process. Connecting with one's core Self is becoming an achievable goal. And with that comes a connection to the whole—a realization that each person makes a difference. Energy moves, and affects that it touches. Everyone expresses energy—both psychically and physically—which has a ripple effect. We can choose what sort of energy we put out.

Achieving balance requires taking the time to care for yourself, as we have suggested throughout these pages. You may need to take steps to restore a badly damaged liver, or build a strong immune system. During the first few months of recovery, an addict's glandular function, nutritional status, nervous system and blood sugar levels are in a very fragile state. Regular nourishing and balanced meals are crucial, as is consistent use of nutritional supplements. Patience is required: no one can redress a lifetime of metabolic imbalance in a week.

Self nurturing means eating well, taking the time to prepare good, wholesome food and *not* obeying the impulse to run to the corner for a quick fast food fill-up. It means walks, time to meditate, pray, or simply listen to soft music. It means time out from the rat race, making contact with and listening to your inner self. It may mean letting go of some parasitic "friends," and spending more alone time. Or, if you tend to isolate, it may mean making new friends and getting out more.

In many cases, a change in environment, including finding supportive friends, relationships and employment situations, can be critical factors for ensuring recovery. Even the hardcore addict can achieve recovery and a new life, as centers such as Delancey Street Foundation, Daytop and Betty Ford Center have shown.

In the initial stages of recovery, you may experience feelings of hopelessness, unworthiness, wild self-destructive impulses, and seemingly uncontrolable rages as you try to break out of the prison of cravings. These kinds of pressures can hurl one back into the spiral of using. The challenge is to find the strength, faith and integrity to grow past this stage and create your new being, with a stable metabolism and lifestyle. Learn to live moderately while not falling into the old trap of overdoing it when you feel good and burning yourself out again. This is part of developing self-love.

When we become whole, self-loving beings, conscious of our deep inner connections to the universe, we enable relationships that are not "needy," but overflow with our own abundance. Then we reach out and touch others with the gift of life. And we truly participate—not endlessly taking from others to fill the void within—but genuinely sharing our love in relationships with others.

Life then becomes the delicious entree: complete, nurturing and bounteous, requiring nothing more, but offering satisfaction. Our relationships become the dessert: the icing on the cake, something to relish and enjoy and devote delighted attention to—they are there simply for the joy of giving and connecting. For the Self is contained and at the same time free.

Many people abuse drugs and alcohol in an attempt to experience happiness. Perhaps the greatest challenge and ultimate fulfillment is finding freedom within ourselves, to accept ourselves and feel the joy that arises from appreciating and knowing life within creation.

You are largely responsible for the creation of your circumstances. Only you can decide to make changes. Once you make that decision, empowerment comes. Learning to be true to yourself can be a major life lesson. Embrace it and allow self-love to surface and be nurtured.

Endnotes to Chapter 13

1. See *The Aquarian Conspiracy*, by Marilyn Ferguson.
2. This is not restricted to the New Age Movement by any means. A significant example is the action groups being formed in many crack-infested ghetto communities. No longer willing to sit back and wait for government action, concerned citizens are taking on the drug dealers. They are organizing block patrols and demonstrations to get them out of their neighborhoods, and reaching out to local officials, demanding not only a crack-down on crack, but jobs for kids, and other measures—in an effort to achieve health, welfare and dignity. (See *Time* and *Newsweek*, September 11, 1989 for special coverage on the crack war.)

Sources Of Help

National Council On Alcoholism

This is an excellent information and referral service which counsels all types of substance abuse clients, including alcoholics, and their loved ones on the various treatment centers, practitioners, educational groups and other support systems available to help them in their recovery process. There is a chapter in every city, although the name can vary slightly as they are a loose association. For more information or to locate the chapter nearest you, call 1-800-NCA-CALL.

Alcoholics Anonymous

Local chapters and meetings of Alcoholics Anonymous can be found in nearly every town and city in the United States and every major city in the western world. The telephone book lists phone numbers for the local chapters, and meeting times, dates, and locations are listed in local newspapers. The national address and phone number are: AA World Services, Box 459, Grand Central Station, New York, NY 10163 (212) 686-1100.

Narcotics Anonymous

Based on the same principles and 12-step program as AA, Narcotics Anonymous meetings are a place substance abusers can go to find real support, inspiration and guidance in the recovery process. Check the telephone directory or newspaper, or call your local chapter of Alcoholics Anonymous for information about meetings in your area.

Co-Dependents Anonymous

Also based on the same principles and 12-step program as AA, Co-Dependents Anonymous meetings support and guide co-dependents in their recovery process. Contact Co-Dependents Anonymous, Inc., International Service Office, Box 33577, Phoenix, AZ 85067-3577, (602) 277-7991 for local meetings.

Treatment Centers

Following are some of the clinics and hospitals that work with holistic methods. Not all of them use the nutritional therapies presented in this book. Contact them first and inquire about the kind of treatment program you are looking for.

Alternatives In Medicine
1200 Tower Building
7th Avenue and Olive Way
Seattle, WA 98101
(206) 467-1818

John Bastyr College
144 N.E. 54th Street
Seattle, WA 98105
(206) 523-9585

Comprehensive Medical Care
76 Louden Avenue
Amityville, NY 11701
(516) 789-7000

Coral Ridge Hospital
Inpatient:
4545 N. Federal Highway
Fort Lauderdale, FL 33308
(305) 771-2711 Ex. 202
Outpatient:
2000 N.E. 47th Street
Fort Lauderdale, FL 33308
(305) 771-2711 Ex. 245

Daytop
Administrative Headquarters
54 West 40th Street
New York, NY 10018
1-800-2-Daytop (24 Hours)

Daytop
631 Woodside Rd.
Redwood City, CA 94061
(415) 367-9030

Delancey Street Foundation
2563 Divisadero
San Francisco, CA 94115
(415) 563-5326 (Days)
(415) 386-1373 (Nights)

Betty Ford Center
39000 Bob Hope Drive
Rancho Mirage, CA 92270
1-800-392-7540 (California
   Only)
1-800-854-9211 (Out of State)

**Haight Ashbury Free
Medical Clinic**
Education Office
409 Clayton Street
San Francisco, CA 94117
(415) 431-1714

Merritt Peralta Institute
435 Hawthorne Ave.
Oakland, CA 94609
(415) 652-7000

**Natural College of
Naturopathic Medicine**
11231 Southeast Market St.
Portland, Oregon 07216
(503) 255-4860

Recovery Systems
147 Lomita Drive
Suite D
Mill Valley, CA 94941
(415) 383-3611

3HO Super Health
2545 North Woodland Rd.
Tucson, AZ 85749
(602) 749-0404

For a complete coverage of drug-alcohol treatment centers in the United States, see *Rehab* by Stan Hart, Harper & Row, New York, 1988.

Sources of Formulas

There are many good companies producing nutritional formulas. I have listed a few of the best so that the unfamiliar reader can have some direction on how to obtain the products discussed in this book. My deepest apologies to those companies not listed herein, but simple limitation of space prevent their acknowledgement. Listing all the good companies would take up an entire book in itself.

A word of caution, however. The nutrition and health food industry (like any other) is rife with companies producing poor quality and even health damaging formulas. There is a great deal of false advertising and misleading information on the effects of products. I urge the reader to be careful in pursuing fad diets and the exaggerated claims of many companies. While there is much that is of value, there is also much that is misrepresented and harmful. Whenever one is dealing with addiction or illness, it is strongly recommended that one seek out the help of a qualified holistic health practitioner.

Vitamins and Minerals

Allergy Research
Amni
Ethical Nutrients
Jarrow Formulas
KAL
Leading Edge Nutrition
Lifestar
Megafood
Metagenics
Mezotrace
Now Vitamins
Probiologic
Rainbow Light
Scientific Consultants
Schiff
SISU
Solgar
Source Natural
Standard Process
Sunrider International
Thompson
Twin Lab

Flax Seed Oil

Allergy Research
Flora
Galaxy Enterprises
Leading Edge Nutrition
Now Vitamins
Omega Nutrition
Omega Nutrition/Arrowhead
   Mills
Probiologic
SISU
Solgar

Standard Process
Threshold

Western Herbs

Amni
Bio Botannica
Ethical Nutrients
Frontier Herbs
Great Health
Herb Pharm
Indiana Botannic Gardens
Jarrow Formulas
Leading Edge Nutrition
Lifestar
Matol
Metagenics
Nature's Way
Phyto-Pharmica
Planetary Formulas
Probiologic
Rainbow Light
Satori
SISU
Standard Process
Sunrider International
Yerba Prima

Chinese Herbs

Bio Botannica
Ethical Nutrients-Metagenics
Herb Pharm
Jarrow Formulas
Leading Edge Nutrition
Nature's Way
Planetary Formulas
Satori
Sunrider International

Ayurvedic Formulas
Leading Edge Nutrition
Planetary Formulas
SISU

Beneficial Intestinal Flora
Allergy Research
Ethical Nutrients
Jarrow Formulas

Leading Edge Nutrition
Lifestar
Metagenics
Probiologic
SISU
Source Naturals
Sunrider International
Yerba Prima

Some Wholesale Sources Of Formulas

Allergy Research
Box 489
San Leadro, CA 94577
1-800-545-9960

Arrowhead Mills/OmegaFlo
Box 2059
Hereford, TX 79045
1-800-733-3744
Fax: (806) 364-8242

Ethical Nutrients-Metagenics
23180 Del Lago
Laguna Hills, CA 92653
(800) 692-9400

Flora, Inc.
Box 950
Lynden, WA 98264
(206) 354-2110
(800) 446-2110

Flora, Inc.
7400 Fraser Park Dr.
Burnaby, B.C.
Canada V5J 5B9

Frontier Herbs
Box 299
Norway, IA 52318
(319) 227-7991
Fax: (319) 227-7966

Galaxy Enterprises, Ltd.
11423-37 B Avenue
Edmonton, Alberta
Canada T6J OK2
(403) 437-7330

Great Health
2663 Saturn St.
Brea, CA 92621
(714) 996-8600

Indiana Botanic Gardens, Inc.
P.O. Box 5
Hammond, IN 46325
(219) 931-2480

Jarrow Formulas
1824 South Robertson Blvd.
Los Angeles, CA 90035
(213) 204-6936
(800) 726-0886
Fax: (213) 204-2520

Leading Edge Nutrition
20 Sunnyside Avenue
Suite A180
Mill Valley, CA 94941
(415) 389-4080

Matol Botanical International
1111 46th Avenue, Suite 100
Lachine, Quebec
Canada H8T 3C5
(514) 639-0730
(800) 363-1890
(800) 383-0162 (in Quebec)

Omega Nutrition
309-8495 Ontario St.
Vancouver, B.C.
Canada V5X 3E8
(604) 322-8862
(800) 661-3529
Fax: (604) 327-2932

Probiologic
1803 132nd Ave. NE
Bellevue, WA 98005
(800) 678-8218
Fax: (206) 882-0771

San Francisco Herb and
  Natural Food Company
1010 46 St.
Emeryville, CA 94608
(800) 523-5192 (CA)
(800) 227-2830 (U.S.)

Satori Teas
401 Ingalles Street
Suite 8
Santa Cruz, CA 95060
(800) 444-7286

SISU Enterprises Ltd.
312-8495 Ontario Street
Vancouver, B.C.
Canada V5X 3E8
(800) 663-4163
(604) 322-6690
Fax: (604) 322-6790

Source Naturals
23 Janis Way
Scotts Valley, CA 95066
(408) 438-6851
(800) 776-7701

Standard Process
Box 38
Campbell, CA 95009-0038
(800) 662-9134

Sunrider International
3111 Lomita Blvd.
Torrance, CA 90505
(213) 534-4786
Fax: (213) 530-4826

Threshold Distributors
P.O. Box 533
Soquel, CA 95073
(800) 438-1700

Yerba Prima
P.O. Box 2569
Oakland, CA 94614
(415) 632-7477

Recommended Reading

Ackerman, R.J., **Children of Alcoholics: Bibliography and Resource Guide** 3rd Edition, Florida: Health Communications, 1983

Airola, Paavo, **Hypoglycemia: A Better Apprach**, Arizona: Health Plus, 1977-Breakthrough work which provided the first medical understanding of this condition. Includes a practical understanding of the importance of diet in treatment.

Al-Anon Family Group, **Al-Anon's Twelve Steps & Twelve Traditions**, New York: Al-Anon Family Group Headquarters, 1981-A thoughtful interpretation of each step and tradition from several viewpoints. Also a story reflecting the practical application of each. This book is used in many step study groups.

Al-Anon: Is It For You?, New York: Al-Anon Family Group Headquarters, 1983

Al-Anon Faces Alcoholism, New York: Al-Anon Family Group Headquarters, 1977

Alcoholics Anonymous World Services, **Alcoholics Anonymous "The Big Book"** 3rd Edition, New York: AA World Services, 1976-The "Bible" of AA. Contains step-by-step guide to recovery from alcoholism. Has facilitated millions of people throughout the world in achieving sobriety and serenity from a disease that previously was thought to be hopeless and incurable.

Appleton, Nancy, Ph.D., **Lick The Sugar Habit**, New York: Avery, 1988-This book provides the most comprehensive understanding of sugar addiction and the deleterious effects of sugar. It includes a self-help program to lick the sugar habit and live a healthier life.

Bates, Charles, Ph.D., **Essential Fatty Acids and Immunity in Mental Health**, Washington: Life Sciences Press, 1987-Excellent Book with recent information on Omega 6 Fatty Acids, GLA, and prostaglandins. Good information on food allergies and alcoholism.

Beattie, Melodie, **Codependent No More—How To Stop Controlling Others and Start Caring for Yourself**, New York: Harper/Hazelden, 1987-This New York Times bestseller is among the very best books on co-dependency, explaining what it is and enumerating the characteristics in a comprehensive checklist as well as explanations of behaviors and how to overcome them.

Cituk, Kathy, and Finnegan, John, **Natural Foods and Good Cooking**, California: Elysian Arts, 1989-Seeing the need for a practical guide to good nutrition, the authors have assembled some of the most valuable and up-to-date inforamtion in an easy-to-use form. Included is information on the Omega 3 fatty acids, cholesterol, butter & oils, salt, the healing properties of various foods and spices, and a variety of easy-to-prepare, delicious recipes.

Cohen, Sidney, M.D.,**The Chemical Brain: The Neurochemistry of Addictive Disorders**, Minneapolis, MN: Care Institute, 1988. A brilliant summary of the latest scientific knowledge in neurochemistry and addiction. The legacy of our formost researcher into the biochemical basis of addictions.

Conrad, Barnaby, **Time Is All We Have**, New York: Dell, 1986-
Honest and inspiring story of the author's four weeks at
the Betty Ford Center. Very warm, human, and acclaimed
as one of the best books on alcohol addiction.

Duffy, William, **Sugar Blues**, Colorado: Warner Books, 1975-
Looking 15 years younger after kicking the sugar habit,
Duffy reveals how the insidious poison invades and destroys lives. His research is excellent. Also how to live
without sugar, including recipes.

Finnegan, John, **Regeneration Of Health**, California: Elysian
Arts, 1989-Provides an in-depth understanding of regeneration through the use of Chinese herbal formulas.

Finnegan, John, **Understanding Oils and Fats**, California, Elysian Arts, 1990 The most complete and up-to-date information on oils and fats in health and disease.

Finnegan, John, **Yeast Disorders**, California: Elysian Arts, 1989-
Provides a comprehensive understanding of this pervasive condition, which is implicated in a number of illnesses including allergies, immune system disorders, liver
dysfunction, skin rashes and faulty digestion. Gives rec-
ommendations on diet and herbal formulas for recovery.

Ford, Betty, with Chase, Chris, **Betty: A Glad Awakening**, New
York: Jove, 1988-The former First Lady shares her battle
with alcoholism and drug addiction and the joy of helping others. A very honest, touching and inspiring story
written straight from the heart.

Friends In Recovery, **The 12 Steps—A Way Out**, California:
Recovery Publications, 1987-A working guide for Adult
Children from addictive and other dysfunctional families.
Utilizes the Twelve Steps as a powerful tool for individu-
als who are seeking to identify and resolve painful issues
from their childhoods.

Gordon, Barbara, **I'm Dancing As Fast As I Can**, New York:
Harper and Row, 1979-The personal "heart-wrenching"
account of one woman's recovery from valium addiction.

Hamaker, John D., **The Survival of Civilization**, California:
Hamaker-Weaver, 1982-Classic work. The original work

on greenhouse effect, global warming, soil depletion, nutritional deficiencies and physical and mental health.

Hay, Louise L., **You Can Heal Your Life**, California: Hay House, 1984-By clearing mental blocks and learning to love and accept ourselves, much illness can be healed. The author shares her first-hand experience of curing herself of terminal cancer, and helps the reader discover and use his or her creative powers to attain health.

Hughs, Richard, and Brewin, Robert, **The Tranquilizing Of America**, New York: Warner Books, 1979

Johnson, Vernon E., **I'll Quit Tomorrow—A Practical Guide To Alcoholism Treatment**, New York: Harper and Row, 1973-This book is used extensively in chemical dependency programs. Good coverage of all facets of intervention and recovery from alcohol abuse *except* nutritional; focusing on physical, mental, psychological and spiritual aspects.

Ketcham, Katherine and Mueller, L. Ann, M.D., **Eating Right To Live Sober**, New York: Writers House, 1983

Langer, Stephen E., **Solved: The Riddle Of Illness**, Connecticut: Keats, 1984-Hypothyroidism can be a contributing factor in many illnesses, including addictions. This little understood condition is elucidated in this well-written work which provides a clear understanding of the gland's function and a simple self-test which can indicate its activity. Thyroid therapy has helped millions of people improve their health and quality of life.

Larsen, Earnie, **Stage II Recovery**, New York: Harper and Row, 1986-Introduces idea that making relationships work is at the heart of full recovery from addictions.

Larsen, Earnie, **Stage II Relationships-Love Beyond Addiction**, New York: Harper and Row, 1987-Clear and practical techniques for couples and families who face the issue of addiction and are striving to bring health and vitality to their lives.

Melodie, Pia, **Facing Co-Dependence-What It is, Where It Comes From, How It Sabotages Our Lives**—Traces the origins of co-dependency back to childhood and describes a range of abuses: physical, sexual, intellectual, spiritual, and emotional.

Milam, James, Dr. and Ketcham, Katherine, **Under The Influence**, New York: Bantam, 1981

Peck, Scott, **The Road Less Travelled—A New Psychology of Love, Traditional Values and Spiritual Growth**, New York: Simon & Schuster, 1978-This Best Seller by a practicing psychiatrist discusses ways of confronting and resolving life's major problems: The working through suffering and pain, gaining wisdom and clarity, ascending to higher levels of consciousness and discovering the spiritual self.

Phelps, Janice Keller, M.D. and Nourse, Alan E., M.D., **The Hidden Addiction And How To Get Free**, Massachusetts: Little, Brown & Co., 1986- Excellent book based on real experience and research.

Reid, Daniel P., **Chinese Herbal Medicine**, Massachusetts: Shambala, 1987

Schaef, Anne Wilson, **Co-Dependence: Misunderstood-Mistreated**, California: Harper & Row, 1986-Defines co-dependence as another form of "the addictive process," which is supported by society. Discusses the impact of this theory on the fields of mental health, chemical dependency, family therapy, and the women's movement.

Schaef, Anne Wilson, **When Society Becomes An Addict**, California: Harper & Row, 1987-New York Times Bestseller. The role of society in promoting and perpetuating addiction.

Schaef, Anne Wilson, **The Addictive Organization**, California: Harper & Row, 1988-Deals succinctly with dysfunctional and addictive systems in business or any other group endeavor—revealing how the addictive system operates, how to recognize it and how to begin the recovery process. Defines workaholism as an addiction fostered by society. Amazing insights. Very inspiring.

Schaef, Anne Wilson, **Escape From Intimacy**, California: Harper & Row, 1989-Exposes and examines the problem of addictions to sex, romance, and relationships. Where does healthy activity end and addiction begin. Describes addictions through their stages.

Schauss, Alexander G., **Diet, Crime and Delinquency**, California: Parker House, 1981-Excellent book by one of the country's foremost authorities in the field.

Schmid, Ronald F., Dr., **Traditional Foods Are Your Best Medicine**, New York: Ballantine, 1987-Researchers have found that many cultures living on traditional foods were free of debilitating diseases. When processed foods were introduced, the population quickly developed diseases common to western culture. Gives good information on the healing properties of foods and provides suggestions for adapting traditional foods into the diet.

Siegel, Bernie, M.D., **Love, Medicine, & Miracles**, New York: Harper & Row, 1986-Unconditional love can stimulate the immune system and heal any illness. Patients find the courage to love themselves enough to allow their bodies to heal. This is one of the most beautiful and inspiring books on healing.

Subby, Robert, **Lost In The Shuffle—The Codependent Reality**, Florida: Health Communications, 1987-Help for the co-dependent to sever the bonds of a troubled past and heal current addictions to the "rules" co-dependents live by.

Sunshine, Linda and Wright, John W., **The 100 Best Treatment Centers For Alcoholism And Drug Abuse**, Avon Books-An excellent guide to the most outstanding Rehabilitation facilities in the country.

Teeguarden, Ron, **Chinese Tonic Herbs**, New York: Japan Publication, 1984

Tierra, Michael, C.A., N.D. **Planetary Herbology**, New Mexico: Lotus Press, 1988

Tierra, Michael, C.A., N.D., **The Way Of Herbs**, New York: Pocket Books, 1983

Treben, Maria, **Health From God's Garden**, Vermont: Healing Arts, 1988

Treben, Maria, **Health Through God's Pharmacy**, Austria: Wilhelm Ennsthaler, Steyr, 1987 - Beautiful book showing the healing uses of common herbs with many case histories.

Verney, Thomas M.D., with Kelly, John, **The Secret Life Of The Unborn Child**, New York: Dell, 1981-The fetus recognizes its mother's feelings and attitudes. It knows if it is wanted or not. Mother's crises, diet (including smoking, drinking, drug-taking), anxieties and joys, all have profound effects on the unborn—which in turn affect that child's self-perception and ability to be in the world.

Whitfield, Charles L., M.D., **Alcholism, Attachments & Spirituality— A Transpersonal Approach**, New Jersey: Distributed by Thomas W. Perrin, Inc., 1985-This self-published work offers an indepth view of the addictive process at work. Seeing a connection between alcoholism and chemical dependence and people's need for attachment to "the way things ought to be," Whitfield discusses how to use suffering as a "gift" and springboard to health, wholeness and spirituality.

Whitfield, Charles L., M.D., **Healing The Child Within—Discovery And Recovery For Adult Children Of Dysfunctional Families**, Florida: Health Communications, 1987-Especially useful for those in the process of recovery from a troubled or dysfunctional family. Defines different forms of abuse, shame, lack of boundaries, co-dependence, compulsion, etc.; how to recognize and heal these syndromes.

Whitfield, Charles L., M.D., **A Gift To Myself: A Personal Workbook and Guide For Healing My Child Within**, Florida: Health Communications, 1990-Dr. Whitfield describes more deeply and in more detail how to heal our child within; i.e., how to do adult child and co-dependency recovery.

Williams, Roger J., Alcoholism: **The Nutritional Approach**, New York: Univ. of Texas Press, 1959

Wilson, Bill, **Alcoholics Anonymous**, New York: 1957

Woititz, Janet, and Geringer, Ed D., **Struggle For Intimacy**, Florida: Health Communications, 1985-With chapters like,

"Who Do You Pick for Your Lover?" "Fear of Loss of Self," "Fear of Abandonment," "Anger," "Trust," "Boundaries," "Expectations," "Loyalty," etc., this book helps co-dependents understand the process they are in and how to climb out of it.

Woititz, Janet, and Geringer, Ed D., **Adult Children Of Alcoholics**, Florida: Health Communications, 1983

Woititz, Janet, and Geringer, Ed D. **Marriage On The Rocks**, Florida: Health Communications, 1979

Wren, R.C., F.L.S., **Potter's New Cyclopaedia of Botanical Drugs and Preparations**, Great Britain: C.W. Daniel Co. Ltd., 1988 - A classic work that has been updated to include information on the pharmacological ingredients and medical properties of herbs.

Yoder, Barbara, **The Recovery Resource Book**, New York: Simon & Schuster, 1990. This excellent book gives a comprehensive survey of recovery resources.

Magazines

Changes—For And About Adult Children, Florida: Health Communications, Inc., - Excellent magazine especially for ACA's but also very relevant for co-dependents or other people from dysfunctional families.

The U.S. Journal Of Drug And Alcohol Dependence, Florida: Health Communications, Inc.

Bibliography

Abel, Ernest L., **Fetal Alcohol Syndrome and Fetal Alcohol Effects**, New York: Research Institute on Alcoholism, 1984

Al-Anon, **One Day At a Time In Al-Anon**, New York: Al-Anon Family Group Hdqtrs., 1987

Alberts, Bruce, et al, **Molecular Biology of The Cell**, Second Edition, New York: Garland Publishing, Inc. 1989

Alcoholics Anonymous World Services, **Twelve Steps and Twelve Traditions**, New York: AA, 1953

Appleton, Nancy, Ph.D., **Lick The Sugar Habit**, New York: Avery, 1988

Barkie, Karen E., **Fancy, Sweet & Sugarfree**, New York: St. Martin's, 1985

Barnes, Broda O., M.D., and Galton Lawrence, **Hypothyroidism: The Unsuspected Illness**, New York: Harper & Row, 1976

Bates, Charles, Ph.d., **Essential Fatty Acids and Immunity in Mental Health**, Washington: Life Sciences Press, 1987

Beasley, Joseph D., M.D., **Wrong Diagnosis, Wrong Treatment**, New York: Creative Informatics, 1987

Beattie, Melody, **Codependent No More**, New York: Harper & Row, 1987

Beck, Deva, R.N., and Beck, James, R.N., **The Pleasure Connection**, CA: Synthesis, 1987

Berry, Carmen Renee, **"The Messiah Trap,"** New Age Journal, Boston: March/April 1987

Bliznakov, Emile G., M.D., and Hunt, Gerald L., **The Miracle Nutrient Coenzyme Q10**, New York: Bantam, 1987

Castine, Jacqueline, **Recovery From Rescuing**, Florida, Health Communications, Inc., 1989

Chishti, Hakim G.M., N.D., **The Traditional Healer**, Vermont: Healing Arts Press, 1988

Cituk, Kathy, and Finnegan, John, **Natural Foods and Good Cooking**, California: Elysian Arts, 1989

Cohen, Sidney, M.D., **The Substance Abuse Problems**, New York: Haworth Press, 1981

Conrad, Barnaby, **Time Is All We Have**, New York: Dell, 1986

Coulart, Frances, **The Caffeine Book**, New York: Dodd Mead & Co., 1984

Cunningham, Donna, MSW, Ramer, Andrew, **The Spiritual Dimensions of Healing Addictions**, California: Cassandra Press, 1988

Dardis, Tom, **The Thirsty Muse**, New York: Ticknor & Fields, 1989

Drug Abuse Survey Project, **Dealing With Drug Abuse —A Report to the Ford Foundation**, New York: Praeger, 1972

Finnegan, John, **Regeneration Of Health**, California: Elysian Arts, 1989

Finnegan, John, **Yeast Disorders**, California: Elysian Arts, 1989

Finnegan, John, **Understanding Oils and Fats**, California: Elysian Arts, 1990

Ford, Betty, with Chase, Chris, **Betty: A Glad Awakening**, New York: Jove, 1988

Fox, Arnold, M.D., and Fox, Barry, **DLPA**, New York: Pocket Books, 1985

Fredericks, Carlton, Ph.D., **Psycho-Nutrition**, New York: Berkley Books, 1988

Fuller, John Grant, **200,000,000 Guinea Pigs**, New York: G.P. Putnam's Sons, 1972

Gitlow, Stanley E., M.D., and Peyser, Herbert S., M.D. Editors, **Alcoholism A Practical Treatment Guide**, Pennsylvania: Grune & Stratton, 1988

Gittleman, Ann Louise, M.S., **Beyond Pritikin**, New York: Bantam, 1988

Gennis, Robert B., **Biomembranes Molecular Structure and Function**, New York: Springer-Verlag, 1989

Graham, Judy, **Evening Primrose Oil**, New York: Thorsons, 1984

Graham, Judy, and Odent Michel, Dr., **The Z Factor**, Vermont: Thorsons, 1986

Gravitz, Herbert, and Bowden, Julie, **Guide to Recovery— A Book For Adult Children Of Alcoholics**, Florida: Learning Publications, Inc., 1985

Griggs, Barbara, Green Pharmacy, **A History of Herbal Medicine**, New York: Viking Press, 1982

Haas, Elson M., M.D., **Staying Healthy with the Seasons**, Berkeley, CA: Celestial Arts, 1981.

Hall, Lindsey, and Cohn, Leigh, **Recoveries**, California: Gurze Books, 1987

Hamaker, John D., **The Survival Of Civilization**, California: Hamaker-Weaver, 1982

Hart, Stan, **Rehab: A Comprehensive Guide to Recommended Drug-Alcohol Treatment Centers in the United States**, New York: Harper & Row, 1988

Hatterer, Lawrence, M.D., **The Pleasure Addicts—The Addictive Process—Food, Sex, Drugs, Alcohol, Work, and More**, New York: A.S. Barnes & Co., 1980

Hay, Louise L., **You Can Heal Your Life**, California: Hay House, 1984

Hazelden Foundation, **The Twelve Steps Of Alcoholics Anonymous**, New York: Harper/Hazelden, 1987

Heinerman, John, **Heinerman's Encyclopedia of Fruits, Vegetables and Herbs**, New York: Parker Publishing Co., 1988

Hoehling, A.A., **The Great Epidemic**, Massachusetts: Little, Brown & Co., 1961

Hoffer, Abram, M.D.,Ph.D., **Orthomolecular Medicine For Physicians**, Connecticut: Keats, 1989

Hughes, Richard, and Brewin, Robert, **The Tranquilizing Of America**, New York: Harcourt Brace Janovich, 1979

Jeffries, William McK., M.D., F.A.C.P., **Safe Uses of Cortisone**, Illinois: Charles C. Thomas, 1981

Keck, Robert L., **The Spirit Of Synergy— God's Power and You,** Tennessee: Parthenon Press, 1978

Ketcham, Katherine and Mueller, L.Ann, M.D., **Eating Right To Live Sober,** New York: Writers House, 1983

Kirschmann, John D. and Dunne, Lavon J., **Nutrition Almanac,** New York: McGraw-Hill, 1984

Langer, Stephen E., M.D., **Solved: The Riddle Of Illness,** Connecticut: Keats, 1984

Lennard & Epstein, **Mystification And Drug Misuse,** California: Jossey-Bass, Inc., 1971

Leonard, Linda Schierse, **Witness To The Fire,** Massachusetts, Shambala, 1989

Mabey, Richard, **The New Age Herbalist,** New York: Collier Books, 1988

Manahan, William, M.D., **Eat For Health,** California: H.J. Kramer, 1988

Milam, James, Dr. and Ketcham, Katherine, **Under The Influence— A Guide To The Myths And Realities Of Alcoholism,** New York: Bantam, 1981

Moore, Richard D., M.D., Ph.D. and Webb, George, Ph.D., **The K Factor,** New York: Pocket Books, 1986

Murray, Dr. Michael, N.D., **The 21st Century Herbal,** Washington: Vita-Line Inc.

Myers, Judy, Ph.D., **Staying Sober,** New York: Pocket Books, 1987

Newbold, H.L., M.D., **Mega-Nutrients For Your Nerves,** New York: Peter H. Wyden, 1975

Page, Melvin E., D.D.S. and Abrams, H. Leon, Jr., **Your Body Is Your Best Doctor!,** Connecticut, Keats, 1972

Peele, Stanton with Brodsky, Archie, **Love and Addiction,** New York: Signet, 1976

Pelton, Ross, R., Ph.D., **Mind Food and Smart Pills,** T & R Publishers, 1986

Pfeiffer, Carl C. Ph.D., M.D. **Nutrition and Mental Illness,** Vermont: Healing Arts, 1987

Pfeiffer, Carl C. Ph.D., M.D., **Zinc And Other Micronutrients,** Connecticut: Keats, 1978

Phelps, Janice Keller, M.D. and Nourse, Alan E., M.D., **The Hidden Addiction And How To Get Free**, Massachusetts: Little, Brown & Co., 1986

Prevention Magazine, **New Encyclopedia Of Common Diseases**, Pennsylvania: Rodale, 1984

Prevention Magazine Editors, **The Complete Book Of Vitamins**, Pennsylvania: Rodale, 1984

Quillin, Patrick, Ph.D., R.D. **Healing Nutrients**, New York: Vintage, 1989

Reid, Daniel P., **Chinese Herbal Medicine**, Massachusetts: Shambala, 1987

Robbins, John, **Diet For A New America**, New Hampshire: Stillpoint, 1987

Rodale, J.I., and Staff, **The Complete Book Of Minerals For Health**, Pennsylvania: Rodale

Rorabaugh, W.J., **The Alcoholic Republic—An American Tradition**, New York: Oxford University Press, 1979

Rudin, Donald O., M.D., and Felix, Clara, **The Omega 3 Phenomenon**, New York: Rawson Associates, 1987

Sabbag, Robert, **Snow Blind,** New York: Avon, 1976

Schaef, Anne Wilson, "We're A Nation Of Addicts," **NewAge Journal**, Boston, March/April, 1987

Schaef, Anne Wilson, **When Society Becomes An Addict**, California: Harper & Row, 1987

Schaef, Anne Wilson, and Fassel, Diane, **The Addictive Organization**, New York: Harper & Row, 1988

Schauss, Alexander G., **Orthomolecular Treatment of Criminal Offenders**, California: Michael Lesser, M.D., 1978

Schauss, Alexander G., **Diet, Crime and Delinquency**, California: Parker House, 1981

Schmid, Ronald F., Dr., **Traditional Foods Are Your Best Medicine**, New York: Ballantine, 1987

Schneider, Meir, **Self Healing, My Life And Vision**, new York: Routledge & Kegan Paul, 1987

Seymour, Richard B. and Smith, David E., M.D., **Drugfree**, New York: Sarah Lazin Books, 1987

Siegel, Bernie, M.D., **Love, Medicine & Miracles**, New York: Harper & Row, 1986

Stoff, Jesse A., M.D. and Pellegrino, Charles R., Ph.D., **Chronic Fatigue Syndrome**, New York: Random House, 1988

Stone, Fromme & Kagan, **Cocaine Seduction And Solution**, New York: Clarkcon, Potter, 1984

Teeguarden, Ron, **Chinese Tonic Herbs**, New York: Japan Publication, 1984

Thomsen, Robert, **Bill Wilson**, New York: Harper & Row, 1975

Tierra, Michael, C.A., N.D., **Planetary Herbology**, New Mexico: Lotus Press, 1988

Tierra, Michael, C.A., N.D., **The Way Of Herbs**, New York: Pocket Books, 1983

Treben, Maria, **Health Through God's Pharmacy**, Austria: Wilhelm Ennsthaler, Steyr, 1987

Treben, Maria, **Health From God's Garden**, Vermont: Healing Arts, 1988

Truss, C. Orian, M.D., **The Missing Diagnosis**, Alabama: C. Orian Truss, M.D., 1985

Weiss, Roger D., M.D., and Mirin, Steven M., M.D., **Cocaine**, Washington DC: American Psychiatric Press, Inc., 1987

Weissman, Joseph D., M.D., **Choose to Live**, New York: Penguin Books, 1988

Werbach, Melvyn R., M.D. **Nutritional Influences On Illness**, California: Third Line Press, 1987

Wren, R.C., F.L.S., **Potter's New Cyclopaedia of Botanical Drugs and Preparations**, Great Britain: C.W. Daniel Co. Ltd., 1988

Young, Klein, Beyer, **Recreational Drugs**, New York: Collier Books, 1977

Zi, Nancy, **The Art Of Breathing**, New York: Bantam, 1986

Index

A

AA (Alcoholics Anonymous), 4–5, 83, 84, 92, 211
Abnormal chemicals, 72–74
Abravanel, Elliot, 109
Acetaminophen (Tylenol), 18
Acetylaldehyde, 24, 72–73
Acidophilus, 142
Action Caps, 122–123
Activity, 81–82
Acupressure, 88
Acupuncture, 87–88
Addictions
  advertising's encouraging of, 6–57
  causes of, 41–49, 61–77
  inner child and, 51–59
  nutritional therapies for, 95–156
  overview of, 1–10
  predisposition to, 52, 56, 57–58
  society's encouraging of, 56–57
  types of, 17–40
  See also Co-dependence; Recovery or specific addiction
Adibi, Siamak, 101
Adrenal glands, 65–67, 109
Adult Child of Alcoholics Anonymous, 84
Advertising, encourages addiction, 56–57
Aerobic exercise, 83
Aftercare, 86–87
Al-Anon, 15, 84, 92
Ala-teen, 84

Ala-tot, 84
Alcohol, addiction to, 23–26, 41
Alcoholic Clinic at Craig Dunaine Hospital (Inverness), 116–117
Alcoholic Republic, The (Rorabaugh), 24
Alcoholics Anonymous (AA), 4–5, 83, 84, 92, 211
Alienation, 44
Allergies, food, 37–38, 152
Allergy Research (San Leandro, CA), 217
Alpha 20C, 124
Alpha-linolenic acid, 70, 103–107, 158–159
Alpha methylfentanyl, 27
Alternatives In Medicine (Seattle, WA), 212
American Indians, 26
American Psychiatric Association, Annual Meeting of, 19
Amino acids, 138–139
Amphetamines, addiction to, 33
Anabolic steroids, 36
"Annie", case history of, 52–56, 58
Antibiotics, 62
Arrowhead Mills/OmegaFlo (Hereford, TX), 159, 217
  flax seed oil of, 107
  oils of, 106
Ascorbic acid, 70, 73, 139–140
Aspirin, 19
Ayurvedic formulas, 217

233

Hypothyroidism: The Unsuspected Illness (Barnes), 66, 121

I
"Ice", 92
IgC Antibody Test, 152
Illich, Ivan, 44, 109
Illness, causes of, 6, 109
"Imperial professions", 44
Inca Empire, 34
Incest Survivors Anonymous, 84
Indiana Botanic Gardens, Inc. (Hammond, IN), 217
Indians (American), 26
Inner child, 51–59, 177–178
In-patient programs, 86–87
International Conference on Pharmacological Treatments for Alcoholism (London), 117
Intestinal flora, beneficial, 142–143, 217
Invalidation, 51, 55–56
Iron, 135–136
Italians, 25

J
Jagger, Mick, 42
Jarrow Formulas (Los Angeles, CA), 218
beneficial digestive flora of, 143
herb teas of, 111
"Jean" (therapist), 189
Jefferson, Thomas, 25
Jeffries, William, 66
"Jerry", case history of, 54–55, 56, 58
John Bastyr College (Seattle, WA), 212
Juices, carrot, celery, and beet, 108
Jung, Carl, 4

K
Kal, nutritional yeast of, 99
"Kathy" (sister), 194
Keller, Janice, 139
"Ken", case history of, 181–182
Kerouac, Jack, 42
Kesey, Ken, 42
Kleber, Herbert, 2–3
Kloss, Jethro, 128
Km, 129–130
Kodak, 69
Kola nut, 31
Korean white ginseng, 118
Korenman, Stanley, 5

L
Lamb Stew, recipe for, 164–165
Langer, Stephen, 13, 66, 121, 125–126
Leading Edge Nutrition (Mill Valley, CA), 218
Lewis Labs, nutritional yeast of, 99
Libby, 139–140
Life Extension, 23
Lifestar, 102
iron of, 136
multiple mineral formula of, 134
Lifestream, 124
Linoleic acid, 70, 103–107, 158–159
Linus Pauling Institute Of Science and Medicine, 137
Liv.52, 7–8, 70, 73, 112–115
Liver
cirrhosis of, 6
damage to, 6–7, 63
function of, 62–65
Liver & Onions, recipe for, 166
"Liza", case history of, 56, 58
Lofentanil, 27

About The Authors

John Finnegan was born in Greenwich Village and raised in Long Island, the jungles of Latin America, and the beaches and redwoods of Northern California. He began writing his first book when he was nine years old—the story of his family's journey from New York to Lima Peru. They were the first people to drive the length of Central America, often having to cut their own road through the jungle with machetes, shovels, and pick-axes.

At nineteen, he began to research the biochemical basis of physical and mental illness, which included studying and work-ing with many of this century's leading medical pioneers. He studied life sciences and social sciences at San Francisco State University, College of Marin, and continued his studies with Dr. John Christopher, Dr. Michael Barnett, Piro Caro, other holistic researchers, and in several medical centers. John Finnegan is the author of six books, including *Amazake*, which he co-authored with Kathy Cituk. He lectures and conducts seminars, and gave presentations at both the 1987 and 1988 San Francisco Whole Life Expos. This book is the culmination of a lifetime of research and work.

Daphne Gray was raised in Topanga Canyon, California, the third of four children. She returned to school after raising four children, travelling to Europe and Cuba, living in Mexico, Kenya, Tanzania, and Angola, and working various jobs, including 10 years as manager of an in-house publisher. She earned her B.A. in Journalism at San Francisco State University in 1983.

Having been raised in an alcoholic home, she has found great sustance in ACA and Coda 12-Step programs. In addition to writing and editing, Daphne works with Chinese herbs and practices body therapy, integrating body/mind acupressure and bioenergetics.

To dance is Daphne's greatest joy. Other interests include Taoist practices, natural healing, health and nutrition, trans-personal psychology and spirituality.

More books that can help from Celestial Arts:

Healing the Addictive Mind by Lee Jampolsky, Ph.D.

The first book to use lessons from *A Course in Miracles* as a tool for overcoming addictive behaviors, including chemical dependency and codependent relationships. Includes daily exercises for overcoming harmful patterns and gaining spiritual peace. *$9.95 paper, 172 pages*

How Shall I Live? by Richard Moss, M.D.

A medical doctor and alternative healthcare advocate discusses how to deal with a major health crisis and how to transform the experience into an opportunity for greater aliveness. Covers issues such as fear, guilt, helplessness, and despair and shows how to release and share your healing energies. *$8.95 paper, 180 pages*

Love Is Letting Go of Fear by Gerald Jampolsky, M.D.

The lessons in this extremely popular little book (over 1,000,000 in print), based on *A Course in Miracles,* will teach you to let go of fear and remember that our true essence is love. Includes daily exercises. *$7.95 paper or $9.95 cloth, 160 pages*

Unlimit Your Life by James Fadiman, Ph.D.

How to assess and understand the factors holding you back in life, and then set concrete goals and start working towards attaining them in the most effective, life-affirming fashion. *$9.95 paper, 224 pages*

Self Esteem by Virgina Satir

This best-selling book presents an essential credo for the individual in modern society. This classic poem, beautifully illustrated, is a simple and succinct declaration of self worth. *$5.95 paper, 64 pages*

Wellness Workbook by John Travis, M.D. and Regina Ryan

The first contemporary book to use the word "wellness" to describe total health—and still one of the most popular. This updated edition provides a wealth of information and exercises for integrating physical, emotional, intellectual, and spiritual factors to create vibrant, life-long health. *$13.95 paper, 256 pages* A TEN SPEED PRESS BOOK

Choose to Be Healthy by Susan Smith Jones, Ph.D.

The choices we make in life can greatly increase our health and happiness— this book details how to analyze one's choices about food, exercise, thought, work, and play, and then use this information to create a better, healthier life. *$9.95 paper, 252 pages*

Choose to Live Peacefully by Susan Smith Jones, Ph.D.

By nurturing our inner selves and living in personal peace, we can help to bring about global change. In this book, Susan Smith Jones explores the many components of a peaceful, satisfying life—including exercise, nutrition, solitude, meditation, ritual, and environmental awareness—and shows how they can be linked to world peace. *$11.95, 320 pages*

Instinctive Nutrition by Severen Schaeffer

Your body instinctively knows what nutrients it needs and what you should eat to be healthy. This book shows how to overcome centuries of social conditioning and learn to listen to your body's real needs, for health, weight loss, and healing. *$8.95 paper, 224 pages*

It's Not What You Eat but What Eats You by Jack Schwartz

"After seeing what Jack Schwartz can do to/with his body, you've got to be interested in what's going on in his mind."—Richard Bolles, author of *What Color is Your Parachute?*

"What most delights and amazes me in the life, the wisdom, and the teachings of my friend (Jack Schwartz) is the way in which his words so often illuminate for me the sayings of the greatest master."—Joseph Campbell

An exploration of the intense mind/body connection between nutrition and vitality. *$8.95 paper, 182 pages*

Staying Healthy with the Seasons by Elson Haas, M.D.

One of the most popular of the new health books, this is a blend of Eastern and Western medicines, nutrition, herbology, exercise, and preventive healthcare. *$12.95 paper, 252 pages*

Available from your local bookstore or order direct from the publisher. Please include $2.50 shipping and handling for the first book and 50¢ for each additional book. California residents include local sales tax. Write for our free complete catalog of over 400 books and tapes.

CELESTIAL ARTS
Post Office Box 7327
Berkeley, California 94707
For VISA or MasterCard orders, call (510) 845-8414